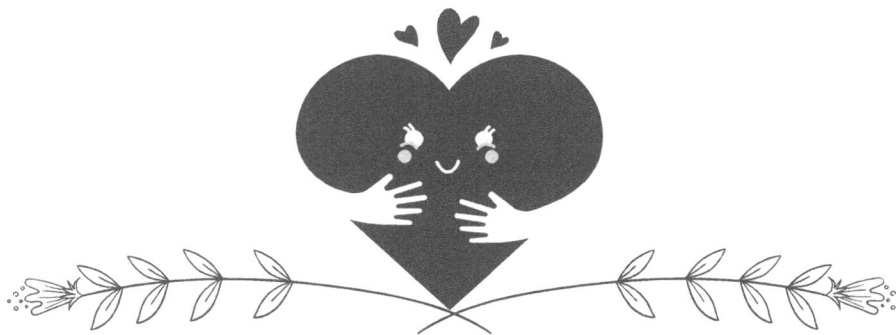

# Blood Pressure
## *LOG BOOK*

**NAME** ————————————————————

**DOB** ————————————————————

**BLOOD TYPE** ————————— **DOCTOR** —————————

**PHONE** ————————————————————

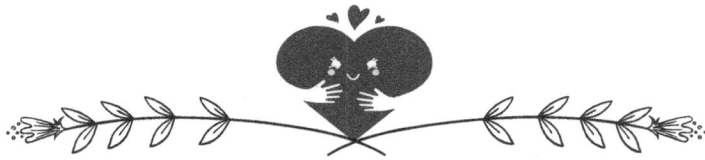

| DATE |  |
|------|--|
| **TIME** |  |
| **SBP** |  |
| **DBP** |  |
| **PULSE** |  |

## DAY_ _ _ _ _ _ _ _ — .

| BLOOD SUGAR | INSULIN DOSE | GRAMS CARB | ACTIVITY |
|-------------|--------------|------------|----------|
|  |  |  |  |
|  |  |  |  |
|  |  |  |  |
|  |  |  |  |

**STRESS LEVELS** _ _ _ _ _ _ _ _ _ _ _ _ _ _ _ _ _

**WATER INTAKE**

## EXERCISE AND DAILY ACTIVITIES

_____

_____

_____

_____

_____

_____

_____

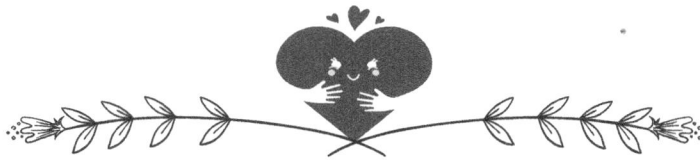

| DATE | |
| TIME | |
| SBP | |
| DBP | |
| PULSE | |

## DAY_ _ _ _ _ _ _ _ .

| BLOOD SUGAR | INSULIN DOSE | GRAMS CARB | ACTIVITY |
|---|---|---|---|
| | | | |
| | | | |
| | | | |
| | | | |

**STRESS LEVELS** _ _ _ _ _ _ _ _ _ _ _ _ _ _ _ _ _ _ _

**WATER INTAKE**

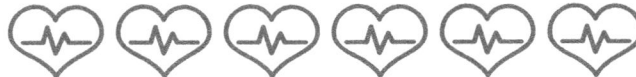

## EXERCISE AND DAILY ACTIVITIES

_____

_____

_____

_____

_____

_____

_____

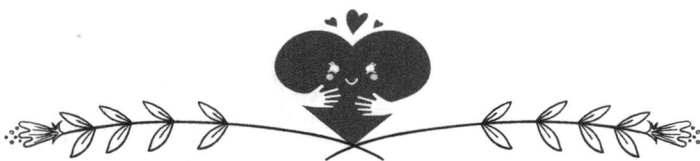

| **DATE** | |
|---|---|
| **TIME** | |
| **SBP** | |
| **DBP** | |
| **PULSE** | |

# DAY_ _ _ _ _ _ _ _ _ .

| BLOOD SUGAR | INSULIN DOSE | GRAMS CARB | ACTIVITY |
|---|---|---|---|
| | | | |
| | | | |
| | | | |
| | | | |

**STRESS LEVELS** _ _ _ _ _ _ _ _ _ _ _ _ _ _

**WATER INTAKE**

## EXERCISE AND DAILY ACTIVITIES

_____

_____

_____

_____

_____

_____

_____

_____

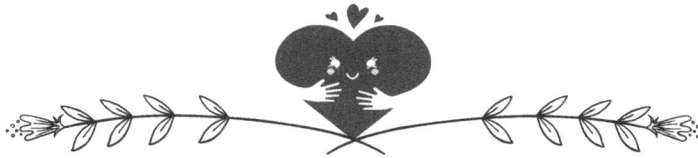

| DATE | |
|---|---|
| **TIME** | |
| **SBP** | |
| **DBP** | |
| **PULSE** | |

## DAY_ _ _ _ _ _ _ _ .

| BLOOD SUGAR | INSULIN DOSE | GRAMS CARB | ACTIVITY |
|---|---|---|---|
| | | | |
| | | | |
| | | | |
| | | | |

**STRESS LEVELS** _ _ _ _ _ _ _ _ _ _ _ _ _ _ _

**WATER INTAKE**

## EXERCISE AND DAILY ACTIVITIES

_____

_____

_____

_____

_____

_____

_____

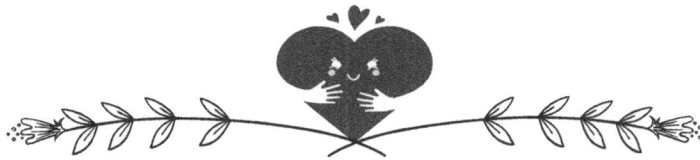

| DATE | |
|------|--|
| **TIME** | |
| **SBP** | |
| **DBP** | |
| **PULSE** | |

## DAY _ _ _ _ _ _ _ _ _ .

| BLOOD SUGAR | INSULIN DOSE | GRAMS CARB | ACTIVITY |
|-------------|--------------|------------|----------|
| | | | |
| | | | |
| | | | |
| | | | |

**STRESS LEVELS** _ _ _ _ _ _ _ _ _ _ _ _ _ _ _

**WATER INTAKE**

## EXERCISE AND DAILY ACTIVITIES

_____

_____

_____

_____

_____

_____

_____

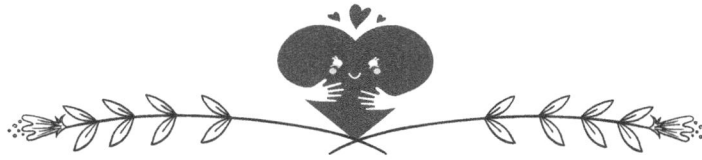

| DATE | |
|------|---|
| TIME | |
| SBP | |
| DBP | |
| PULSE | |

## DAY_ _ _ _ _ _ _ _.

| BLOOD SUGAR | INSULIN DOSE | GRAMS CARB | ACTIVITY |
|-------------|--------------|-----------|----------|
|             |              |           |          |
|             |              |           |          |
|             |              |           |          |
|             |              |           |          |

**STRESS LEVELS** _ _ _ _ _ _ _ _ _ _ _ _ _ _

**WATER INTAKE**

## EXERCISE AND DAILY ACTIVITIES

_____

_____

_____

_____

_____

_____

_____

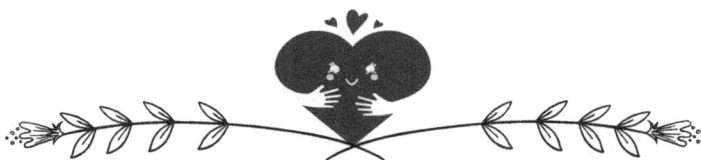

| DATE |  |
|------|--|
| TIME |  |
| SBP |  |
| DBP |  |
| PULSE |  |

## DAY _ _ _ _ _ _ _ _ .

| BLOOD SUGAR | INSULIN DOSE | GRAMS CARB | ACTIVITY |
|-------------|--------------|------------|----------|
|  |  |  |  |
|  |  |  |  |
|  |  |  |  |
|  |  |  |  |

**STRESS LEVELS** _ _ _ _ _ _ _ _ _ _ _ _ _ _

**WATER INTAKE**

## EXERCISE AND DAILY ACTIVITIES

_____

_____

_____

_____

_____

_____

_____

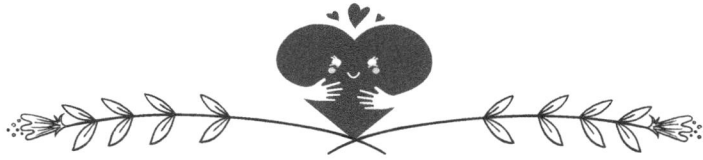

| DATE | |
|------|--|
| **TIME** | |
| **SBP** | |
| **DBP** | |
| **PULSE** | |

## DAY_ _ _ _ _ _ _ _ _ .

| BLOOD SUGAR | INSULIN DOSE | GRAMS CARB | ACTIVITY |
|-------------|--------------|-----------|----------|
| | | | |
| | | | |
| | | | |
| | | | |

**STRESS LEVELS** _ _ _ _ _ _ _ _ _ _ _ _ _ _ _

**WATER INTAKE** ♡ ♡ ♡ ♡ ♡ ♡

## EXERCISE AND DAILY ACTIVITIES

_____

_____

_____

_____

_____

_____

_____

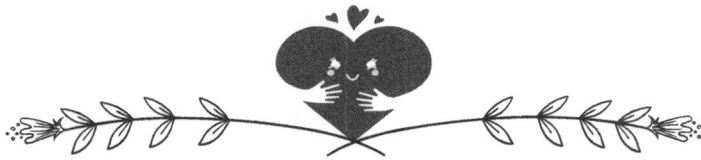

| DATE | |
|------|--|
| **TIME** | |
| **SBP** | |
| **DBP** | |
| **PULSE** | |

## DAY_ _ _ _ _ _ _ _

| BLOOD SUGAR | INSULIN DOSE | GRAMS CARB | ACTIVITY |
|-------------|--------------|-----------|----------|
| | | | |
| | | | |
| | | | |
| | | | |

**STRESS LEVELS** _ _ _ _ _ _ _ _ _ _ _ _ _ _

**WATER INTAKE**

## EXERCISE AND DAILY ACTIVITIES

_____

_____

_____

_____

_____

_____

_____

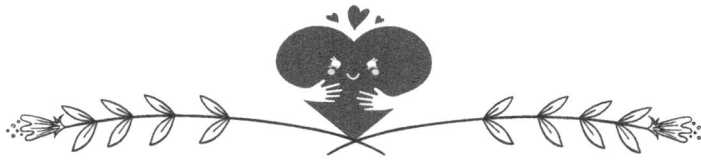

| DATE  |  |
|-------|--|
| TIME  |  |
| SBP   |  |
| DBP   |  |
| PULSE |  |

## DAY_ _ _ _ _ _ _ _ _ .

| BLOOD SUGAR | INSULIN DOSE | GRAMS CARB | ACTIVITY |
|-------------|--------------|------------|----------|
|             |              |            |          |
|             |              |            |          |
|             |              |            |          |
|             |              |            |          |

**STRESS LEVELS** _ _ _ _ _ _ _ _ _ _ _ _ _ _ _ _ _ _ _

**WATER INTAKE**

## EXERCISE AND DAILY ACTIVITIES

_____

_____

_____

_____

_____

_____

_____

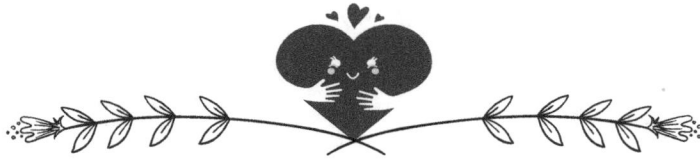

| DATE |  |
|---|---|
| TIME |  |
| SBP |  |
| DBP |  |
| PULSE |  |

# DAY _ _ _ _ _ _ _ .

| BLOOD SUGAR | INSULIN DOSE | GRAMS CARB | ACTIVITY |
|---|---|---|---|
|  |  |  |  |
|  |  |  |  |
|  |  |  |  |
|  |  |  |  |

**STRESS LEVELS** _ _ _ _ _ _ _ _ _ _ _ _ _ _

**WATER INTAKE**

# EXERCISE AND DAILY ACTIVITIES

_____

_____

_____

_____

_____

_____

_____

_____

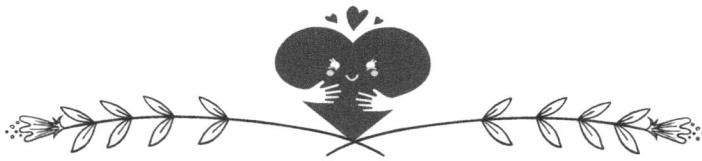

| DATE | |
|------|---|
| **TIME** | |
| **SBP** | |
| **DBP** | |
| **PULSE** | |

# DAY_ _ _ _ _ _ _ _ _ _ .

| BLOOD SUGAR | INSULIN DOSE | GRAMS CARB | ACTIVITY |
|-------------|--------------|-----------|----------|
| | | | |
| | | | |
| | | | |
| | | | |

**STRESS LEVELS** _ _ _ _ _ _ _ _ _ _ _ _ _ _ _

**WATER INTAKE**

## EXERCISE AND DAILY ACTIVITIES

_____

_____

_____

_____

_____

_____

_____

_____

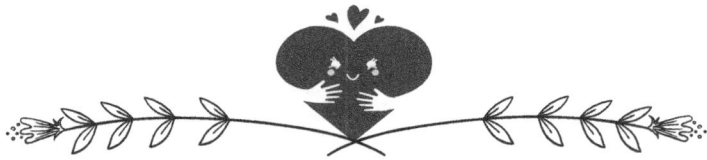

| DATE | |
|------|---|
| TIME | |
| SBP | |
| DBP | |
| PULSE | |

## DAY_ _ _ _ _ _ _ _ .

| BLOOD SUGAR | INSULIN DOSE | GRAMS CARB | ACTIVITY |
|-------------|--------------|------------|----------|
| | | | |
| | | | |
| | | | |
| | | | |

**STRESS LEVELS** _ _ _ _ _ _ _ _ _ _ _ _ _

**WATER INTAKE**  ♡ ♡ ♡ ♡ ♡ ♡

## EXERCISE AND DAILY ACTIVITIES

_____

_____

_____

_____

_____

_____

_____

| DATE | |
| PULSE | |

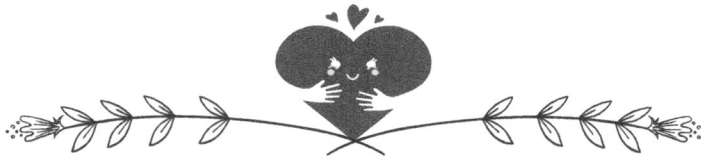

| DATE | |
|---|---|
| TIME | |
| SBP | |
| DBP | |
| PULSE | |

## DAY _ _ _ _ _ _ _ _ _ .

| BLOOD SUGAR | INSULIN DOSE | GRAMS CARB | ACTIVITY |
|---|---|---|---|
| | | | |
| | | | |
| | | | |
| | | | |

**STRESS LEVELS** _ _ _ _ _ _ _ _ _ _ _ _ _ _ _

**WATER INTAKE**

## EXERCISE AND DAILY ACTIVITIES

_____

_____

_____

_____

_____

_____

_____

_____

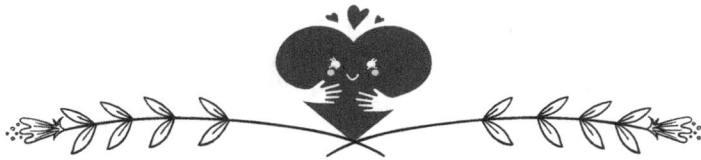

| DATE | |
|------|--|
| TIME | |
| SBP | |
| DBP | |
| PULSE | |

## DAY_ _ _ _ _ _ _ _ .

| BLOOD SUGAR | INSULIN DOSE | GRAMS CARB | ACTIVITY |
|-------------|--------------|-----------|----------|
| | | | |
| | | | |
| | | | |
| | | | |

**STRESS LEVELS** _ _ _ _ _ _ _ _ _ _ _ _ _ _ _ _

**WATER INTAKE**

## EXERCISE AND DAILY ACTIVITIES

_____

_____

_____

_____

_____

_____

_____

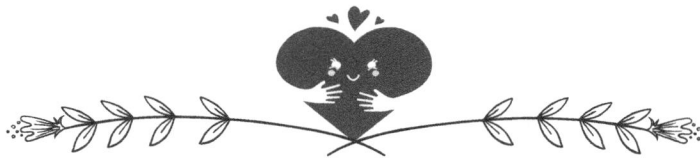

| DATE |  |
|------|--|

| TIME |  |
|------|--|

| SBP |  |
|-----|--|

| DBP |  |
|-----|--|

| PULSE |  |
|-------|--|

## DAY_ _ _ _ _ _ _ _ _ _ .

| BLOOD SUGAR | INSULIN DOSE | GRAMS CARB | ACTIVITY |
|-------------|--------------|------------|----------|
|             |              |            |          |
|             |              |            |          |
|             |              |            |          |
|             |              |            |          |

**STRESS LEVELS** _ _ _ _ _ _ _ _ _ _ _ _ _ _ _ _ _

**WATER INTAKE**

## EXERCISE AND DAILY ACTIVITIES

_____

_____

_____

_____

_____

_____

_____

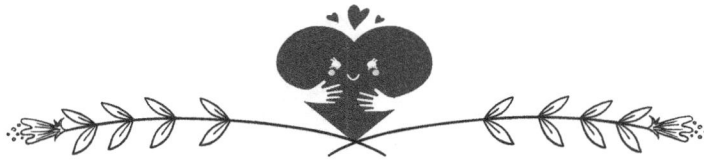

| DATE | |
|------|--|
| TIME | |
| SBP | |
| DBP | |
| PULSE | |

# DAY_ _ _ _ _ _ _ _ _ _ .

| BLOOD SUGAR | INSULIN DOSE | GRAMS CARB | ACTIVITY |
|-------------|--------------|-----------|----------|
| | | | |
| | | | |
| | | | |
| | | | |

**STRESS LEVELS** _ _ _ _ _ _ _ _ _ _ _ _ _ _

**WATER INTAKE**

## EXERCISE AND DAILY ACTIVITIES

_____

_____

_____

_____

_____

_____

_____

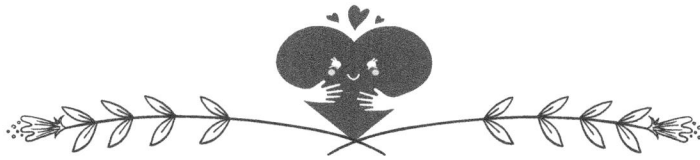

| DATE | |
|------|---|
| **TIME** | |
| **SBP** | |
| **DBP** | |
| **PULSE** | |

## DAY_ _ _ _ _ _ _ _ .

| BLOOD SUGAR | INSULIN DOSE | GRAMS CARB | ACTIVITY |
|-------------|--------------|-----------|----------|
| | | | |
| | | | |
| | | | |
| | | | |

**STRESS LEVELS** _ _ _ _ _ _ _ _ _ _ _ _ _ _

**WATER INTAKE**

## EXERCISE AND DAILY ACTIVITIES

_____

_____

_____

_____

_____

_____

_____

_____

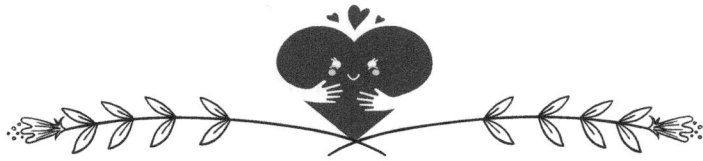

| DATE |  |
|---|---|
| TIME |  |
| SBP |  |
| DBP |  |
| PULSE |  |

# DAY _ _ _ _ _ _ _ _ .

| BLOOD SUGAR | INSULIN DOSE | GRAMS CARB | ACTIVITY |
|---|---|---|---|
|  |  |  |  |
|  |  |  |  |
|  |  |  |  |
|  |  |  |  |

**STRESS LEVELS** _ _ _ _ _ _ _ _ _ _ _ _ _ _ _ _ _

**WATER INTAKE**

## EXERCISE AND DAILY ACTIVITIES

_____

_____

_____

_____

_____

_____

_____

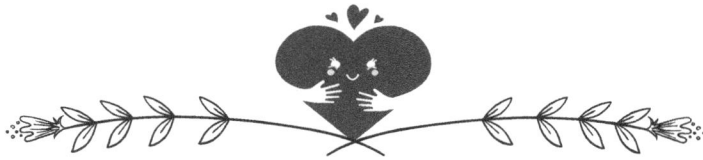

| DATE | |
|------|--|
| **TIME** | |
| **SBP** | |
| **DBP** | |
| **PULSE** | |

## DAY _ _ _ _ _ _ _ _ _ _ .

| BLOOD SUGAR | INSULIN DOSE | GRAMS CARB | ACTIVITY |
|-------------|--------------|------------|----------|
| | | | |
| | | | |
| | | | |
| | | | |

**STRESS LEVELS** _ _ _ _ _ _ _ _ _ _ _ _ _ _ _ _ _ _

**WATER INTAKE**

## EXERCISE AND DAILY ACTIVITIES

_____

_____

_____

_____

_____

_____

_____

_____

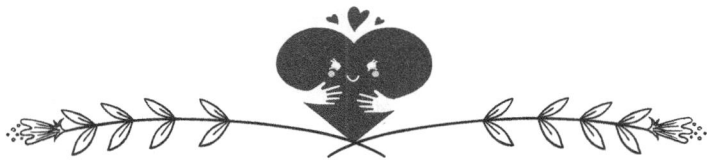

| DATE |  |
|------|--|
| **TIME** |  |
| **SBP** |  |
| **DBP** |  |
| **PULSE** |  |

## DAY _ _ _ _ _ _ _ _ .

| BLOOD SUGAR | INSULIN DOSE | GRAMS CARB | ACTIVITY |
|-------------|--------------|-----------|----------|
|  |  |  |  |
|  |  |  |  |
|  |  |  |  |
|  |  |  |  |

**STRESS LEVELS** _ _ _ _ _ _ _ _ _ _ _ _ _ _

**WATER INTAKE**

## EXERCISE AND DAILY ACTIVITIES

_____

_____

_____

_____

_____

_____

_____

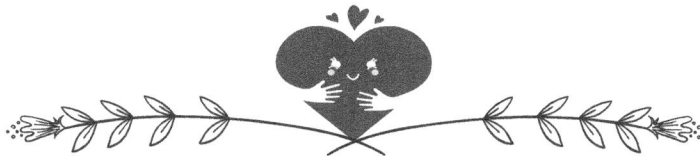

| DATE  |  |
|-------|--|
| TIME  |  |
| SBP   |  |
| DBP   |  |
| PULSE |  |

## DAY _ _ _ _ _ _ _ .

| BLOOD SUGAR | INSULIN DOSE | GRAMS CARB | ACTIVITY |
|-------------|--------------|-----------|----------|
|             |              |           |          |
|             |              |           |          |
|             |              |           |          |
|             |              |           |          |

**STRESS LEVELS** _ _ _ _ _ _ _ _ _ _ _ _ _ _

**WATER INTAKE**

## EXERCISE AND DAILY ACTIVITIES

_____

_____

_____

_____

_____

_____

_____

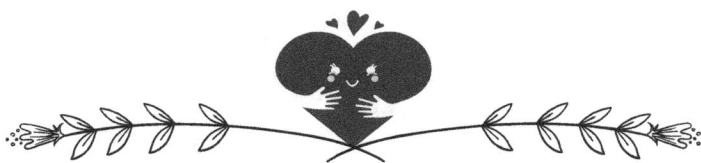

| DATE | |
| --- | --- |
| TIME | |
| SBP | |
| DBP | |
| PULSE | |

## DAY_ _ _ _ _ _ _ .

| BLOOD SUGAR | INSULIN DOSE | GRAMS CARB | ACTIVITY |
| --- | --- | --- | --- |
| | | | |
| | | | |
| | | | |
| | | | |

**STRESS LEVELS** _ _ _ _ _ _ _ _ _ _ _ _ _ _

**WATER INTAKE**

## EXERCISE AND DAILY ACTIVITIES

_____

_____

_____

_____

_____

_____

_____

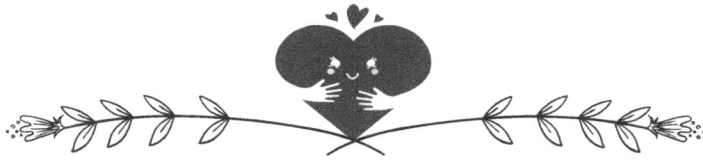

| DATE |  |
| TIME |  |
| SBP |  |
| DBP |  |
| PULSE |  |

## DAY_ _ _ _ _ _ _ _ _.

| BLOOD SUGAR | INSULIN DOSE | GRAMS CARB | ACTIVITY |
|---|---|---|---|
|  |  |  |  |
|  |  |  |  |
|  |  |  |  |
|  |  |  |  |

**STRESS LEVELS** _ _ _ _ _ _ _ _ _ _ _ _ _ _ _ _

**WATER INTAKE**

## EXERCISE AND DAILY ACTIVITIES

_____

_____

_____

_____

_____

_____

_____

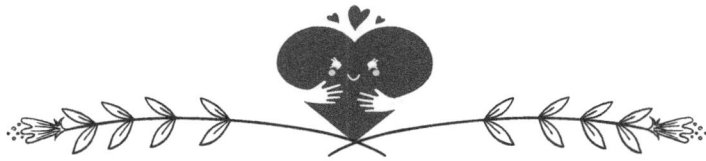

| DATE | |
|---|---|
| **TIME** | |
| **SBP** | |
| **DBP** | |
| **PULSE** | |

## DAY_ _ _ _ _ _ _ _ _ .

| BLOOD SUGAR | INSULIN DOSE | GRAMS CARB | ACTIVITY |
|---|---|---|---|
| | | | |
| | | | |
| | | | |
| | | | |

**STRESS LEVELS** _ _ _ _ _ _ _ _ _ _

**WATER INTAKE**

## EXERCISE AND DAILY ACTIVITIES

_____

_____

_____

_____

_____

_____

_____

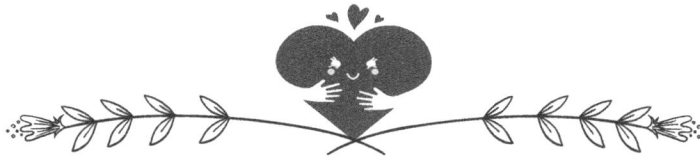

| DATE |  |
|------|--|

| TIME |  |
|------|--|

| SBP |  |
|-----|--|

| DBP |  |
|-----|--|

| PULSE |  |
|-------|--|

## DAY_ _ _ _ _ _ _ _ .

| BLOOD SUGAR | INSULIN DOSE | GRAMS CARB | ACTIVITY |
|-------------|--------------|------------|----------|
|  |  |  |  |
|  |  |  |  |
|  |  |  |  |
|  |  |  |  |

**STRESS LEVELS** _ _ _ _ _ _ _ _ _ _ _ _ _ _

**WATER INTAKE**  ♡ ♡ ♡ ♡ ♡ ♡

## EXERCISE AND DAILY ACTIVITIES

_____

_____

_____

_____

_____

_____

_____

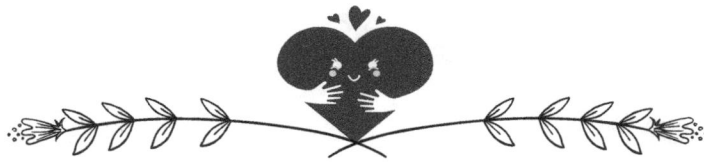

| DATE |  |
|------|--|
| TIME |  |
| SBP  |  |
| DBP  |  |
| PULSE |  |

## DAY _ _ _ _ _ _ _ _ _ .

| BLOOD SUGAR | INSULIN DOSE | GRAMS CARB | ACTIVITY |
|-------------|--------------|-----------|----------|
|             |              |           |          |
|             |              |           |          |
|             |              |           |          |
|             |              |           |          |

**STRESS LEVELS** _ _ _ _ _ _ _ _ _ _ _ _ _

**WATER INTAKE**

## EXERCISE AND DAILY ACTIVITIES

_____

_____

_____

_____

_____

_____

_____

_____

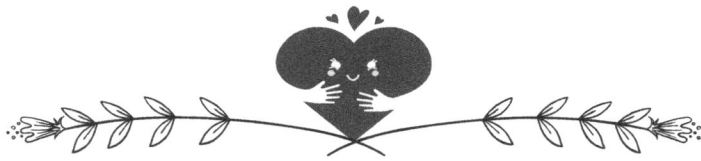

| DATE  |  |
|-------|--|
| TIME  |  |
| SBP   |  |
| DBP   |  |
| PULSE |  |

## DAY_ _ _ _ _ _ _ _ _ _ .

| BLOOD SUGAR | INSULIN DOSE | GRAMS CARB | ACTIVITY |
|-------------|--------------|------------|----------|
|             |              |            |          |
|             |              |            |          |
|             |              |            |          |
|             |              |            |          |

**STRESS LEVELS** _ _ _ _ _ _ _ _ _ _ _ _ _ _ _

**WATER INTAKE**

## EXERCISE AND DAILY ACTIVITIES

_____

_____

_____

_____

_____

_____

_____

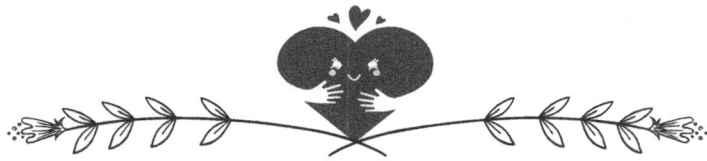

| DATE | |
|---|---|
| **TIME** | |
| **SBP** | |
| **DBP** | |
| **PULSE** | |

## DAY_ _ _ _ _ _ _ _ _ .

| BLOOD SUGAR | INSULIN DOSE | GRAMS CARB | ACTIVITY |
|---|---|---|---|
| | | | |
| | | | |
| | | | |
| | | | |

**STRESS LEVELS** _ _ _ _ _ _ _ _ _ _ _ _ _ _ _

**WATER INTAKE**

## EXERCISE AND DAILY ACTIVITIES

_____

_____

_____

_____

_____

_____

_____

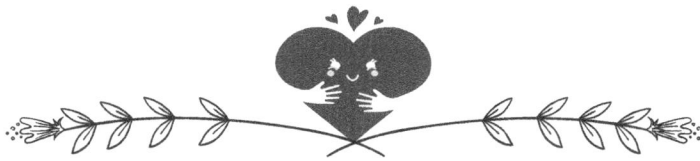

| DATE  |  |
|-------|--|
| TIME  |  |
| SBP   |  |
| DBP   |  |
| PULSE |  |

## DAY_ _ _ _ _ _ _ _ _ .

| BLOOD SUGAR | INSULIN DOSE | GRAMS CARB | ACTIVITY |
|-------------|--------------|------------|----------|
|             |              |            |          |
|             |              |            |          |
|             |              |            |          |
|             |              |            |          |

**STRESS LEVELS** _ _ _ _ _ _ _ _ _ _ _ _ _ _ _

**WATER INTAKE**

## EXERCISE AND DAILY ACTIVITIES

_____

_____

_____

_____

_____

_____

_____

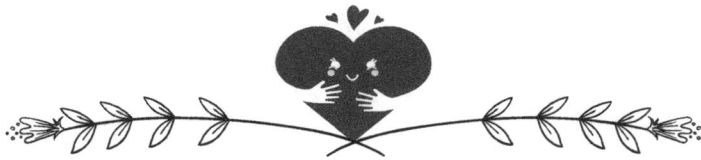

| DATE | |
|------|---|
| **TIME** | |
| **SBP** | |
| **DBP** | |
| **PULSE** | |

## DAY_ _ _ _ _ _ _ _ .

| BLOOD SUGAR | INSULIN DOSE | GRAMS CARB | ACTIVITY |
|-------------|--------------|------------|----------|
| | | | |
| | | | |
| | | | |
| | | | |

**STRESS LEVELS** _ _ _ _ _ _ _ _ _ _ _ _ _ _ _ _ _

**WATER INTAKE**

## EXERCISE AND DAILY ACTIVITIES

_____

_____

_____

_____

_____

_____

_____

_____

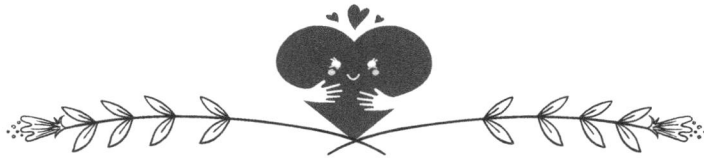

| DATE | |
|------|--|
| **TIME** | |
| **SBP** | |
| **DBP** | |
| **PULSE** | |

# DAY_ _ _ _ _ _ _ _ _ _ .

| BLOOD SUGAR | INSULIN DOSE | GRAMS CARB | ACTIVITY |
|-------------|--------------|------------|----------|
| | | | |
| | | | |
| | | | |
| | | | |

**STRESS LEVELS** _ _ _ _ _ _ _ _ _ _ _ _

**WATER INTAKE**

# EXERCISE AND DAILY ACTIVITIES

_____

_____

_____

_____

_____

_____

_____

_____

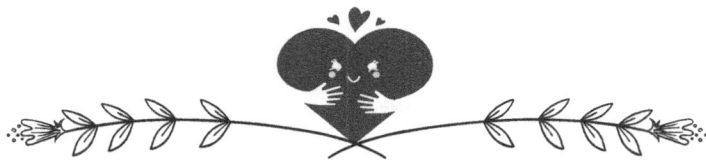

| DATE | |
|------|--|
| **TIME** | |
| **SBP** | |
| **DBP** | |
| **PULSE** | |

## DAY_ _ _ _ _ _ _ _ .

| BLOOD SUGAR | INSULIN DOSE | GRAMS CARB | ACTIVITY |
|-------------|--------------|-----------|----------|
| | | | |
| | | | |
| | | | |
| | | | |

**STRESS LEVELS** _ _ _ _ _ _ _ _ _ _ _ _ _ _

**WATER INTAKE**

## EXERCISE AND DAILY ACTIVITIES

_____

_____

_____

_____

_____

_____

_____

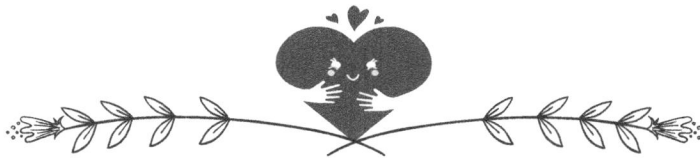

| DATE | |
|------|--|
| **TIME** | |
| **SBP** | |
| **DBP** | |
| **PULSE** | |

## DAY_ _ _ _ _ _ _ _ _ _ .

| BLOOD SUGAR | INSULIN DOSE | GRAMS CARB | ACTIVITY |
|-------------|--------------|-----------|----------|
| | | | |
| | | | |
| | | | |
| | | | |

**STRESS LEVELS** _ _ _ _ _ _ _ _ _ _ _ _ _ _ _ _ _ _

**WATER INTAKE**

## EXERCISE AND DAILY ACTIVITIES

_____

_____

_____

_____

_____

_____

_____

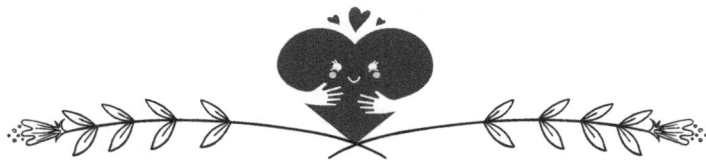

| DATE |  |
|------|--|
| TIME |  |
| SBP |  |
| DBP |  |
| PULSE |  |

## DAY_ _ _ _ _ _ _ _ .

| BLOOD SUGAR | INSULIN DOSE | GRAMS CARB | ACTIVITY |
|-------------|--------------|------------|----------|
|             |              |            |          |
|             |              |            |          |
|             |              |            |          |
|             |              |            |          |

**STRESS LEVELS** _ _ _ _ _ _ _ _ _ _ _ _ _ _ _ _

**WATER INTAKE**

## EXERCISE AND DAILY ACTIVITIES

_____

_____

_____

_____

_____

_____

_____

_____

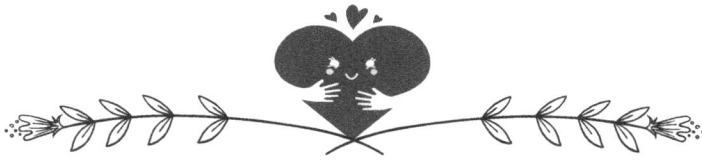

| DATE |  |
|---|---|
| TIME |  |
| SBP |  |
| DBP |  |
| PULSE |  |

# DAY_ _ _ _ _ _ _ _ _ .

| BLOOD SUGAR | INSULIN DOSE | GRAMS CARB | ACTIVITY |
|---|---|---|---|
|  |  |  |  |
|  |  |  |  |
|  |  |  |  |
|  |  |  |  |

**STRESS LEVELS** _ _ _ _ _ _ _ _ _ _ _ _ _ _ _ _

**WATER INTAKE**

## EXERCISE AND DAILY ACTIVITIES

_____

_____

_____

_____

_____

_____

_____

_____

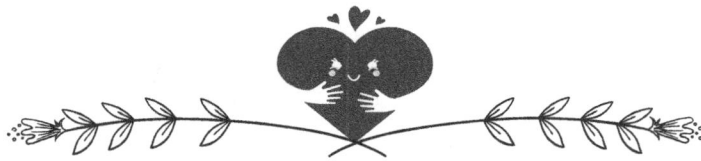

| DATE | |
|------|--|
| TIME | |
| SBP | |
| DBP | |
| PULSE | |

## DAY_ _ _ _ _ _ _ _ .

| BLOOD SUGAR | INSULIN DOSE | GRAMS CARB | ACTIVITY |
|-------------|--------------|------------|----------|
| | | | |
| | | | |
| | | | |
| | | | |

**STRESS LEVELS** _ _ _ _ _ _ _ _ _ _ _ _ _

**WATER INTAKE**

## EXERCISE AND DAILY ACTIVITIES

_____

_____

_____

_____

_____

_____

_____

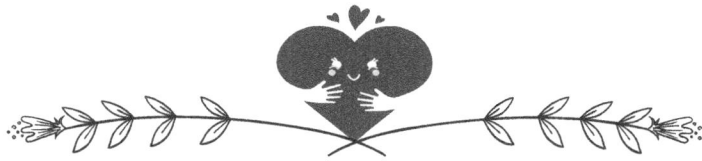

| DATE | |
|------|--|
| **TIME** | |
| **SBP** | |
| **DBP** | |
| **PULSE** | |

## DAY_ _ _ _ _ _ _ _.

| BLOOD SUGAR | INSULIN DOSE | GRAMS CARB | ACTIVITY |
|-------------|--------------|-----------|----------|
| | | | |
| | | | |
| | | | |
| | | | |

**STRESS LEVELS** _ _ _ _ _ _ _ _ _ _ _ _ _ _ _ _ _ _

**WATER INTAKE**

## EXERCISE AND DAILY ACTIVITIES

_____

_____

_____

_____

_____

_____

_____

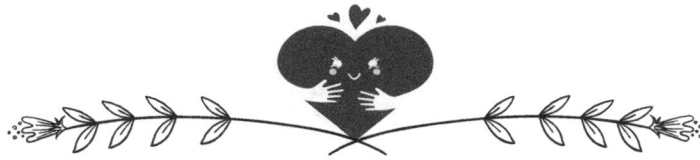

| DATE | |
|---|---|
| TIME | |
| SBP | |
| DBP | |
| PULSE | |

# DAY_ _ _ _ _ _ _ _ _ _ .

| BLOOD SUGAR | INSULIN DOSE | GRAMS CARB | ACTIVITY |
|---|---|---|---|
| | | | |
| | | | |
| | | | |
| | | | |

**STRESS LEVELS** _ _ _ _ _ _ _ _ _ _ _ _ _

**WATER INTAKE**

## EXERCISE AND DAILY ACTIVITIES

_____

_____

_____

_____

_____

_____

_____

_____

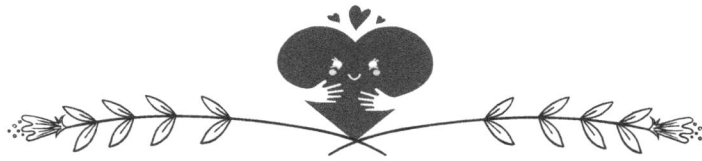

| **DATE** | |
| **TIME** | |
| **SBP** | |
| **DBP** | |
| **PULSE** | |

## DAY_ _ _ _ _ _ _ _ _ _ .

| BLOOD SUGAR | INSULIN DOSE | GRAMS CARB | ACTIVITY |
|---|---|---|---|
| | | | |
| | | | |
| | | | |
| | | | |

**STRESS LEVELS** _ _ _ _ _ _ _ _ _ _ _ _ _ _

**WATER INTAKE**

## EXERCISE AND DAILY ACTIVITIES

_____

_____

_____

_____

_____

_____

_____

_____

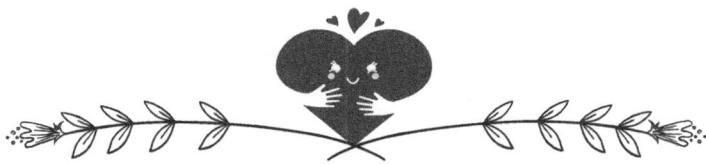

| DATE | |
|---|---|
| **TIME** | |
| **SBP** | |
| **DBP** | |
| **PULSE** | |

# DAY_ _ _ _ _ _ _ _ .

| BLOOD SUGAR | INSULIN DOSE | GRAMS CARB | ACTIVITY |
|---|---|---|---|
| | | | |
| | | | |
| | | | |
| | | | |

**STRESS LEVELS** _ _ _ _ _ _ _ _ _ _ _ _ _

**WATER INTAKE**

## EXERCISE AND DAILY ACTIVITIES

_____

_____

_____

_____

_____

_____

_____

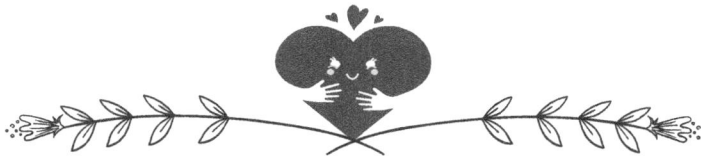

| DATE | |
|------|---|
| **TIME** | |
| **SBP** | |
| **DBP** | |
| **PULSE** | |

## DAY_ _ _ _ _ _ _ .

| BLOOD SUGAR | INSULIN DOSE | GRAMS CARB | ACTIVITY |
|-------------|--------------|-----------|----------|
| | | | |
| | | | |
| | | | |
| | | | |

**STRESS LEVELS** _ _ _ _ _ _ _ _ _ _ _ _ _ _ _ _

**WATER INTAKE**

## EXERCISE AND DAILY ACTIVITIES

_____

_____

_____

_____

_____

_____

_____

_____

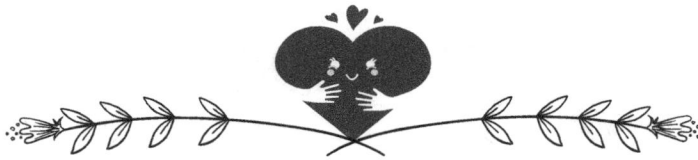

| DATE | |
|---|---|
| TIME | |
| SBP | |
| DBP | |
| PULSE | |

# DAY_ _ _ _ _ _ _ _ .

| BLOOD SUGAR | INSULIN DOSE | GRAMS CARB | ACTIVITY |
|---|---|---|---|
| | | | |
| | | | |
| | | | |
| | | | |

**STRESS LEVELS** _ _ _ _ _ _ _ _ _ _ _ _ _

**WATER INTAKE**

## EXERCISE AND DAILY ACTIVITIES

_____

_____

_____

_____

_____

_____

_____

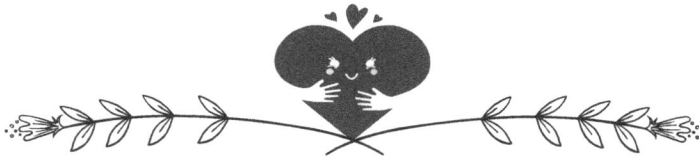

| DATE | |
|---|---|
| TIME | |
| SBP | |
| DBP | |
| PULSE | |

## DAY_ _ _ _ _ _ _ _ _ .

| BLOOD SUGAR | INSULIN DOSE | GRAMS CARB | ACTIVITY |
|---|---|---|---|
| | | | |
| | | | |
| | | | |
| | | | |

**STRESS LEVELS** _ _ _ _ _ _ _ _ _ _ _ _ _ _ _

**WATER INTAKE** ♥ ♥ ♥ ♥ ♥ ♥

## EXERCISE AND DAILY ACTIVITIES

_____

_____

_____

_____

_____

_____

_____

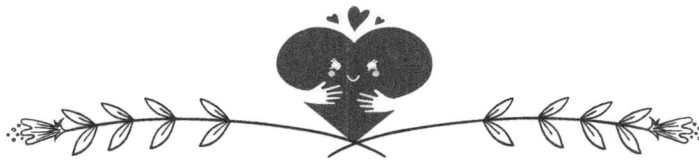

| DATE | |
|------|--|
| **TIME** | |
| **SBP** | |
| **DBP** | |
| **PULSE** | |

## DAY _ _ _ _ _ _ _ _ .

| BLOOD SUGAR | INSULIN DOSE | GRAMS CARB | ACTIVITY |
|-------------|--------------|------------|----------|
|  |  |  |  |
|  |  |  |  |
|  |  |  |  |
|  |  |  |  |

**STRESS LEVELS** _ _ _ _ _ _ _ _ _ _ _ _ _ _ _

**WATER INTAKE**

## EXERCISE AND DAILY ACTIVITIES

_____

_____

_____

_____

_____

_____

_____

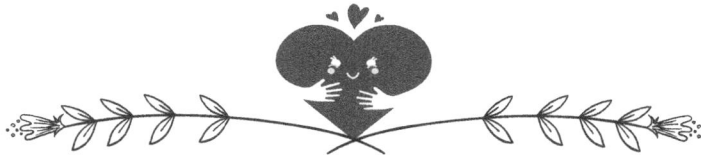

| DATE |  |
|------|--|
| TIME |  |
| SBP |  |
| DBP |  |
| PULSE |  |

## DAY_ _ _ _ _ _ _ _ _ _ _ .

| BLOOD SUGAR | INSULIN DOSE | GRAMS CARB | ACTIVITY |
|-------------|--------------|-----------|----------|
|  |  |  |  |
|  |  |  |  |
|  |  |  |  |
|  |  |  |  |

**STRESS LEVELS** _ _ _ _ _ _ _ _ _ _ _ _ _ _ _ _ _ _

**WATER INTAKE**

## EXERCISE AND DAILY ACTIVITIES

_____

_____

_____

_____

_____

_____

_____

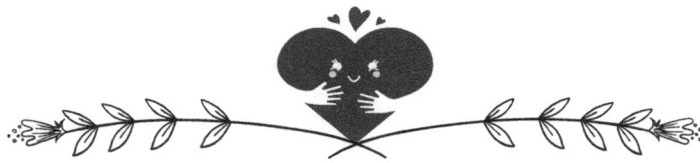

| DATE | |
|------|--|
| TIME | |
| SBP | |
| DBP | |
| PULSE | |

## DAY_ _ _ _ _ _ _ _ _.

| BLOOD SUGAR | INSULIN DOSE | GRAMS CARB | ACTIVITY |
|-------------|--------------|-----------|----------|
| | | | |
| | | | |
| | | | |
| | | | |

**STRESS LEVELS** _ _ _ _ _ _ _ _ _ _ _ _

**WATER INTAKE**

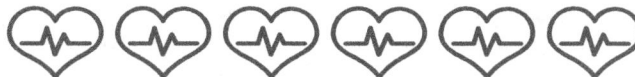

## EXERCISE AND DAILY ACTIVITIES

_____

_____

_____

_____

_____

_____

_____

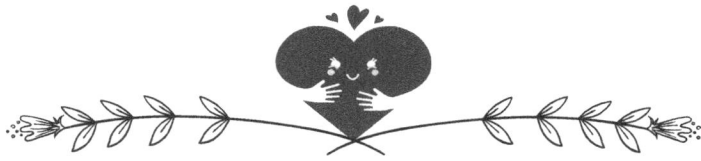

| DATE | |
|------|--|
| **TIME** | |
| **SBP** | |
| **DBP** | |
| **PULSE** | |

# DAY_ _ _ _ _ _ _ .

| BLOOD SUGAR | INSULIN DOSE | GRAMS CARB | ACTIVITY |
|-------------|--------------|------------|----------|
| | | | |
| | | | |
| | | | |
| | | | |

**STRESS LEVELS** _ _ _ _ _ _ _ _ _ _ _ _ _ _ _ _

**WATER INTAKE**

# EXERCISE AND DAILY ACTIVITIES

_____

_____

_____

_____

_____

_____

_____

_____

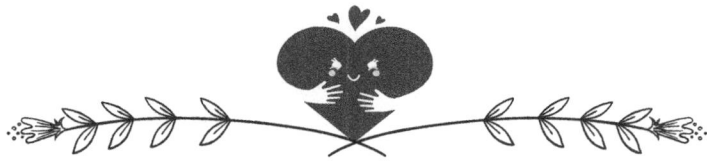

| DATE | |
|------|--|
| **TIME** | |
| **SBP** | |
| **DBP** | |
| **PULSE** | |

## DAY_ _ _ _ _ _ _ _ _ .

| BLOOD SUGAR | INSULIN DOSE | GRAMS CARB | ACTIVITY |
|-------------|--------------|-----------|----------|
| | | | |
| | | | |
| | | | |
| | | | |

**STRESS LEVELS** _ _ _ _ _ _ _ _ _ _ _ _ _

**WATER INTAKE**

## EXERCISE AND DAILY ACTIVITIES

_____

_____

_____

_____

_____

_____

_____

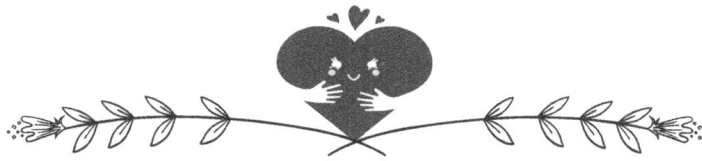

| DATE |  |
|------|--|
| **TIME** |  |
| **SBP** |  |
| **DBP** |  |
| **PULSE** |  |

# DAY_ _ _ _ _ _ _ _ _ _ _ .

| BLOOD SUGAR | INSULIN DOSE | GRAMS CARB | ACTIVITY |
|-------------|--------------|------------|----------|
|  |  |  |  |
|  |  |  |  |
|  |  |  |  |
|  |  |  |  |

**STRESS LEVELS** _ _ _ _ _ _ _ _ _ _ _ _ _ _ _ _ _ _

**WATER INTAKE**

## EXERCISE AND DAILY ACTIVITIES

_____

_____

_____

_____

_____

_____

_____

_____

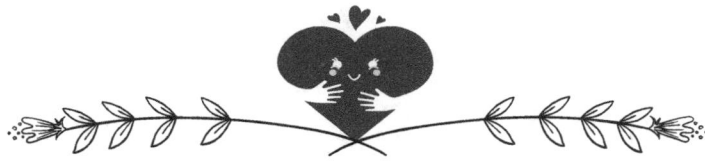

| DATE |  |
|------|--|
| **TIME** |  |
| **SBP** |  |
| **DBP** |  |
| **PULSE** |  |

# DAY_ _ _ _ _ _ _ _ _ _ .

| BLOOD SUGAR | INSULIN DOSE | GRAMS CARB | ACTIVITY |
|-------------|--------------|-----------|----------|
|  |  |  |  |
|  |  |  |  |
|  |  |  |  |
|  |  |  |  |

**STRESS LEVELS** _ _ _ _ _ _ _ _ _ _ _ _ _ _

**WATER INTAKE**

# EXERCISE AND DAILY ACTIVITIES

_____

_____

_____

_____

_____

_____

_____

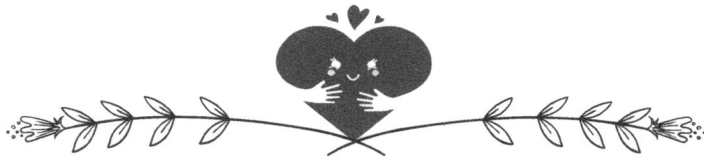

| DATE | |
|------|---|
| **TIME** | |
| **SBP** | |
| **DBP** | |
| **PULSE** | |

## DAY_ _ _ _ _ _ _ _ _ .

| BLOOD SUGAR | INSULIN DOSE | GRAMS CARB | ACTIVITY |
|-------------|--------------|-----------|----------|
| | | | |
| | | | |
| | | | |
| | | | |

**STRESS LEVELS** _ _ _ _ _ _ _ _ _ _ _ _ _ _ _ _ _

**WATER INTAKE**

## EXERCISE AND DAILY ACTIVITIES

_____

_____

_____

_____

_____

_____

_____

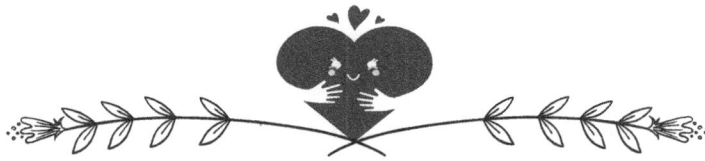

| DATE |  |
|------|--|
| **TIME** |  |
| **SBP** |  |
| **DBP** |  |
| **PULSE** |  |

## DAY_ _ _ _ _ _ _ _ _ .

| BLOOD SUGAR | INSULIN DOSE | GRAMS CARB | ACTIVITY |
|-------------|--------------|------------|----------|
|  |  |  |  |
|  |  |  |  |
|  |  |  |  |
|  |  |  |  |

**STRESS LEVELS** _ _ _ _ _ _ _ _ _ _ _ _ _ _ _

**WATER INTAKE**  ♡ ♡ ♡ ♡ ♡ ♡

## EXERCISE AND DAILY ACTIVITIES

_____

_____

_____

_____

_____

_____

_____

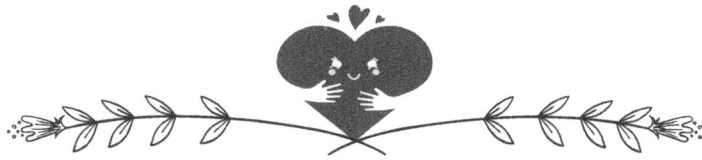

| DATE | |
|---|---|
| TIME | |
| SBP | |
| DBP | |
| PULSE | |

## DAY_ _ _ _ _ _ _ _ .

| BLOOD SUGAR | INSULIN DOSE | GRAMS CARB | ACTIVITY |
|---|---|---|---|
| | | | |
| | | | |
| | | | |
| | | | |

**STRESS LEVELS** _ _ _ _ _ _ _ _ _ _ _ _ _ _ _

**WATER INTAKE**  ♡ ♡ ♡ ♡ ♡ ♡

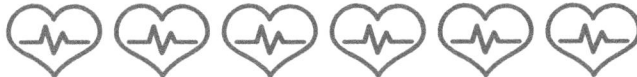

## EXERCISE AND DAILY ACTIVITIES

_____

_____

_____

_____

_____

_____

_____

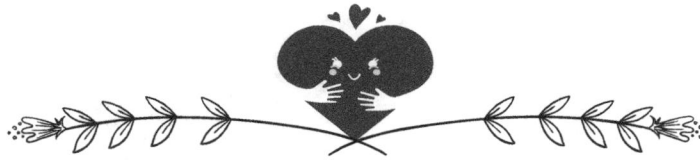

| DATE | |
|------|---|
| **TIME** | |
| **SBP** | |
| **DBP** | |
| **PULSE** | |

## DAY_ _ _ _ _ _ _ _ .

| BLOOD SUGAR | INSULIN DOSE | GRAMS CARB | ACTIVITY |
|-------------|--------------|-----------|----------|
| | | | |
| | | | |
| | | | |
| | | | |

**STRESS LEVELS** _ _ _ _ _ _ _ _ _ _ _ _

**WATER INTAKE**

## EXERCISE AND DAILY ACTIVITIES

_____

_____

_____

_____

_____

_____

_____

_____

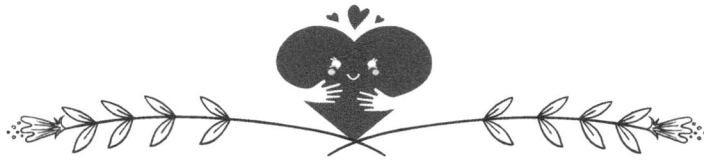

| DATE | |
|------|--|
| **TIME** | |
| **SBP** | |
| **DBP** | |
| **PULSE** | |

## DAY_ _ _ _ _ _ _ _ _ .

| BLOOD SUGAR | INSULIN DOSE | GRAMS CARB | ACTIVITY |
|-------------|--------------|-----------|----------|
| | | | |
| | | | |
| | | | |
| | | | |

**STRESS LEVELS** _ _ _ _ _ _ _ _ _ _ _ _ _ _ _ _

**WATER INTAKE**

## EXERCISE AND DAILY ACTIVITIES

_____

_____

_____

_____

_____

_____

_____

_____

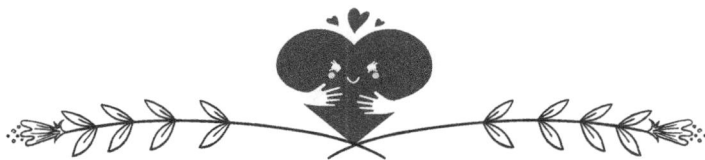

| DATE | |
|---|---|
| TIME | |
| SBP | |
| DBP | |
| PULSE | |

## DAY_ _ _ _ _ _ _ _ _ .

| BLOOD SUGAR | INSULIN DOSE | GRAMS CARB | ACTIVITY |
|---|---|---|---|
| | | | |
| | | | |
| | | | |
| | | | |

**STRESS LEVELS** _ _ _ _ _ _ _ _ _ _ _ _ _ _ _

**WATER INTAKE**

## EXERCISE AND DAILY ACTIVITIES

_____

_____

_____

_____

_____

_____

_____

_____

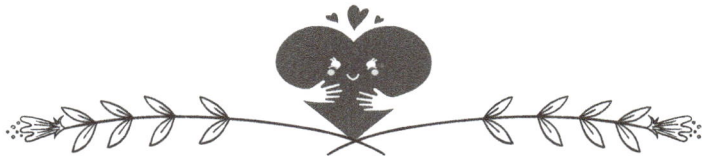

| DATE |  |
|------|--|
| TIME |  |
| SBP |  |
| DBP |  |
| PULSE |  |

## DAY_ _ _ _ _ _ _ _ _ .

| BLOOD SUGAR | INSULIN DOSE | GRAMS CARB | ACTIVITY |
|-------------|--------------|------------|----------|
|             |              |            |          |
|             |              |            |          |
|             |              |            |          |
|             |              |            |          |

**STRESS LEVELS** _ _ _ _ _ _ _ _ _ _ _ _ _

**WATER INTAKE**

## EXERCISE AND DAILY ACTIVITIES

_____

_____

_____

_____

_____

_____

_____

_____

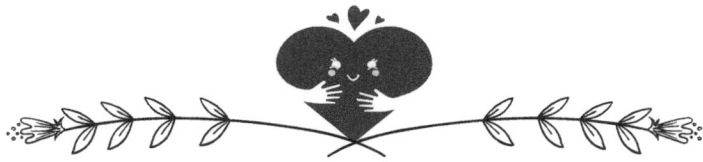

| DATE | |
| TIME | |
| SBP | |
| DBP | |
| PULSE | |

## DAY_ _ _ _ _ _ _ _ _.

| BLOOD SUGAR | INSULIN DOSE | GRAMS CARB | ACTIVITY |
|---|---|---|---|
| | | | |
| | | | |
| | | | |
| | | | |

**STRESS LEVELS** _ _ _ _ _ _ _ _ _ _ _ _ _ _

**WATER INTAKE**   ♡ ♡ ♡ ♡ ♡ ♡

## EXERCISE AND DAILY ACTIVITIES

_____

_____

_____

_____

_____

_____

_____

_____

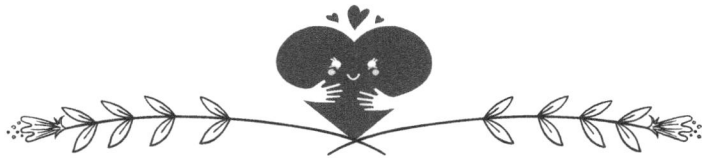

| DATE |  |
|------|--|

| TIME |  |
|------|--|

| SBP |  |
|------|--|

| DBP |  |
|------|--|

| PULSE |  |
|------|--|

## DAY_ _ _ _ _ _ _ _ _ .

| BLOOD SUGAR | INSULIN DOSE | GRAMS CARB | ACTIVITY |
|-------------|--------------|------------|----------|
|  |  |  |  |
|  |  |  |  |
|  |  |  |  |
|  |  |  |  |

**STRESS LEVELS** _ _ _ _ _ _ _ _ _ _ _ _ _ _ _ _

**WATER INTAKE**

## EXERCISE AND DAILY ACTIVITIES

_____

_____

_____

_____

_____

_____

_____

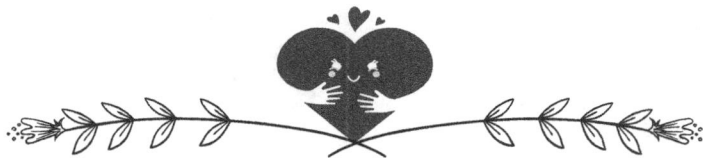

| DATE | |
|---|---|
| **TIME** | |
| **SBP** | |
| **DBP** | |
| **PULSE** | |

## DAY _ _ _ _ _ _ _ _ .

| BLOOD SUGAR | INSULIN DOSE | GRAMS CARB | ACTIVITY |
|---|---|---|---|
| | | | |
| | | | |
| | | | |
| | | | |

**STRESS LEVELS** _ _ _ _ _ _ _ _ _ _ _ _ _ _ _

**WATER INTAKE**

## EXERCISE AND DAILY ACTIVITIES

_____

_____

_____

_____

_____

_____

_____

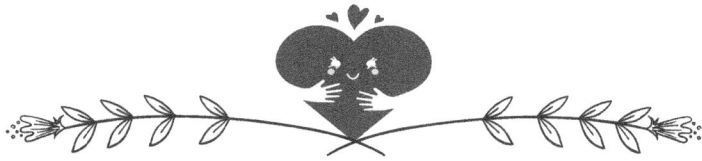

| DATE | |
|---|---|
| TIME | |
| SBP | |
| DBP | |
| PULSE | |

## DAY_ _ _ _ _ _ _ _ .

| BLOOD SUGAR | INSULIN DOSE | GRAMS CARB | ACTIVITY |
|---|---|---|---|
| | | | |
| | | | |
| | | | |
| | | | |

**STRESS LEVELS** _ _ _ _ _ _ _ _ _ _ _ _ _ _ _

**WATER INTAKE**

## EXERCISE AND DAILY ACTIVITIES

_____

_____

_____

_____

_____

_____

_____

_____

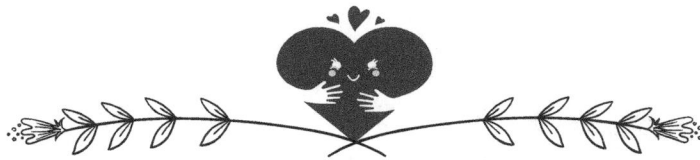

| DATE |  |
|---|---|
| TIME |  |
| SBP |  |
| DBP |  |
| PULSE |  |

## DAY_ _ _ _ _ _ _ _ _ .

| BLOOD SUGAR | INSULIN DOSE | GRAMS CARB | ACTIVITY |
|---|---|---|---|
|  |  |  |  |
|  |  |  |  |
|  |  |  |  |
|  |  |  |  |

**STRESS LEVELS** _ _ _ _ _ _ _ _ _ _ _ _ _

**WATER INTAKE**

## EXERCISE AND DAILY ACTIVITIES

_____

_____

_____

_____

_____

_____

_____

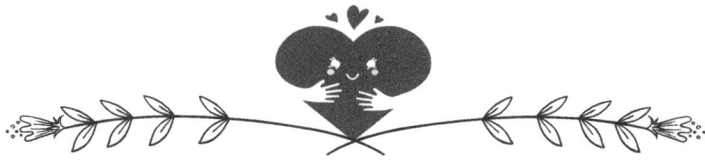

| DATE | |
|------|---|
| **TIME** | |
| **SBP** | |
| **DBP** | |
| **PULSE** | |

## DAY_ _ _ _ _ _ _ _ _ _ .

| BLOOD SUGAR | INSULIN DOSE | GRAMS CARB | ACTIVITY |
|-------------|--------------|------------|----------|
| | | | |
| | | | |
| | | | |
| | | | |

**STRESS LEVELS** _ _ _ _ _ _ _ _ _ _ _ _ _ _ _ _

**WATER INTAKE**

## EXERCISE AND DAILY ACTIVITIES

_____

_____

_____

_____

_____

_____

_____

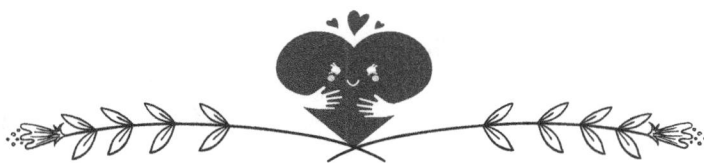

| DATE | |
|------|---|
| TIME | |
| SBP | |
| DBP | |
| PULSE | |

## DAY _ _ _ _ _ _ _ _ .

| BLOOD SUGAR | INSULIN DOSE | GRAMS CARB | ACTIVITY |
|-------------|--------------|-----------|----------|
| | | | |
| | | | |
| | | | |
| | | | |

**STRESS LEVELS** _ _ _ _ _ _ _ _ _ _ _ _

**WATER INTAKE**

## EXERCISE AND DAILY ACTIVITIES

_____

_____

_____

_____

_____

_____

_____

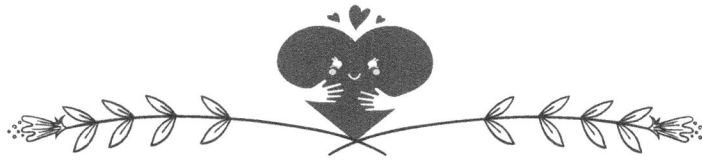

| DATE | |
|------|--|
| **TIME** | |
| **SBP** | |
| **DBP** | |
| **PULSE** | |

## DAY_ _ _ _ _ _ _ .

| BLOOD SUGAR | INSULIN DOSE | GRAMS CARB | ACTIVITY |
|-------------|--------------|-----------|----------|
|             |              |           |          |
|             |              |           |          |
|             |              |           |          |
|             |              |           |          |

**STRESS LEVELS** _ _ _ _ _ _ _ _ _ _ _ _ _ _ _

**WATER INTAKE**

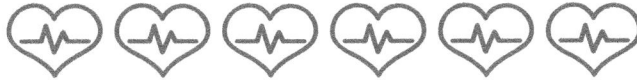

# EXERCISE AND DAILY ACTIVITIES

_____

_____

_____

_____

_____

_____

_____

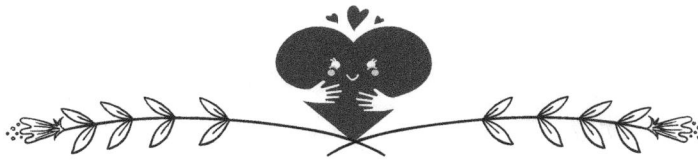

| DATE | |
|---|---|
| TIME | |
| SBP | |
| DBP | |
| PULSE | |

## DAY_ _ _ _ _ _ _ _ .

| BLOOD SUGAR | INSULIN DOSE | GRAMS CARB | ACTIVITY |
|---|---|---|---|
| | | | |
| | | | |
| | | | |
| | | | |

**STRESS LEVELS** _ _ _ _ _ _ _ _ _ _ _ _ _

**WATER INTAKE**

## EXERCISE AND DAILY ACTIVITIES

_____

_____

_____

_____

_____

_____

_____

_____

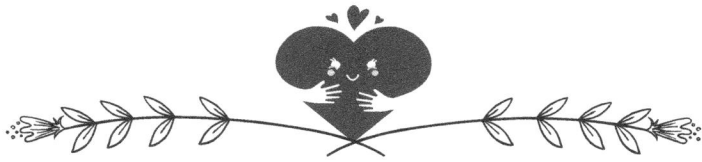

| DATE |  |
|------|--|
| TIME |  |
| SBP |  |
| DBP |  |
| PULSE |  |

## DAY_ _ _ _ _ _ _ .

| BLOOD SUGAR | INSULIN DOSE | GRAMS CARB | ACTIVITY |
|-------------|--------------|------------|----------|
|  |  |  |  |
|  |  |  |  |
|  |  |  |  |
|  |  |  |  |

**STRESS LEVELS** _ _ _ _ _ _ _ _ _ _ _ _ _ _

**WATER INTAKE**

## EXERCISE AND DAILY ACTIVITIES

_____

_____

_____

_____

_____

_____

_____

_____

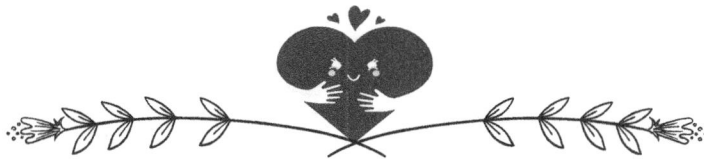

| DATE | |
|------|---|
| **TIME** | |
| **SBP** | |
| **DBP** | |
| **PULSE** | |

## DAY_ _ _ _ _ _ _ _ _ _ .

| BLOOD SUGAR | INSULIN DOSE | GRAMS CARB | ACTIVITY |
|-------------|--------------|------------|----------|
| | | | |
| | | | |
| | | | |
| | | | |

**STRESS LEVELS** _ _ _ _ _ _ _ _ _ _ _ _ _ _ _ .

**WATER INTAKE**

## EXERCISE AND DAILY ACTIVITIES

_____

_____

_____

_____

_____

_____

_____

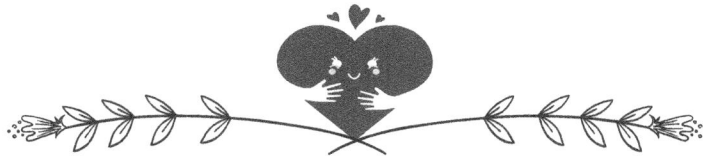

| DATE |  |
|------|--|
| **TIME** |  |
| **SBP** |  |
| **DBP** |  |
| **PULSE** |  |

## DAY_ _ _ _ _ _ _ _ _ .

| BLOOD SUGAR | INSULIN DOSE | GRAMS CARB | ACTIVITY |
|-------------|--------------|-----------|----------|
|  |  |  |  |
|  |  |  |  |
|  |  |  |  |
|  |  |  |  |

**STRESS LEVELS** _ _ _ _ _ _ _ _ _ _ _ _ _ _

**WATER INTAKE**

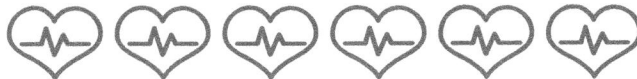

## EXERCISE AND DAILY ACTIVITIES

_____

_____

_____

_____

_____

_____

_____

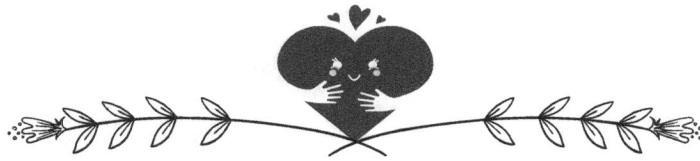

| DATE |  |
|------|--|
| TIME |  |
| SBP |  |
| DBP |  |
| PULSE |  |

## DAY _ _ _ _ _ _ _ _ _ .

| BLOOD SUGAR | INSULIN DOSE | GRAMS CARB | ACTIVITY |
|-------------|--------------|-----------|----------|
|  |  |  |  |
|  |  |  |  |
|  |  |  |  |
|  |  |  |  |

**STRESS LEVELS** _ _ _ _ _ _ _ _ _ _ _

**WATER INTAKE**

## EXERCISE AND DAILY ACTIVITIES

_____

_____

_____

_____

_____

_____

_____

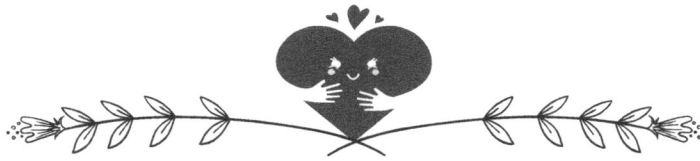

| DATE | |
|------|--|
| **TIME** | |
| **SBP** | |
| **DBP** | |
| **PULSE** | |

## DAY_ _ _ _ _ _ _ _ _ _ .

| BLOOD SUGAR | INSULIN DOSE | GRAMS CARB | ACTIVITY |
|-------------|--------------|-----------|----------|
| | | | |
| | | | |
| | | | |
| | | | |

**STRESS LEVELS** _ _ _ _ _ _ _ _ _ _ _ _ _ _ _

**WATER INTAKE**

## EXERCISE AND DAILY ACTIVITIES

_____

_____

_____

_____

_____

_____

_____

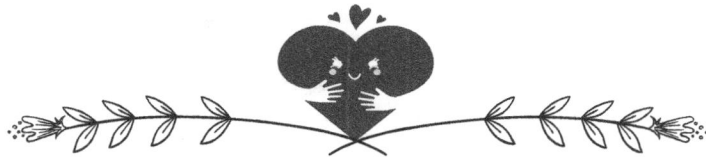

| DATE |  |
|------|--|
| TIME |  |
| SBP |  |
| DBP |  |
| PULSE |  |

## DAY_ _ _ _ _ _ _ _ _ _ .

| BLOOD SUGAR | INSULIN DOSE | GRAMS CARB | ACTIVITY |
|-------------|--------------|------------|----------|
|             |              |            |          |
|             |              |            |          |
|             |              |            |          |
|             |              |            |          |

**STRESS LEVELS** _ _ _ _ _ _ _ _ _ _ _ _ _ _

**WATER INTAKE**  ♡ ♡ ♡ ♡ ♡ ♡

## EXERCISE AND DAILY ACTIVITIES

_____

_____

_____

_____

_____

_____

_____

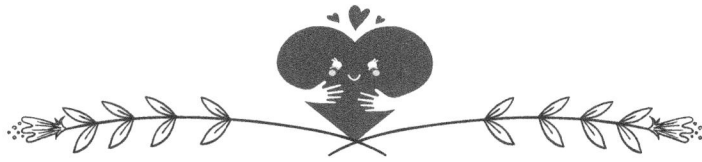

| DATE |  |
|---|---|
| **TIME** |  |
| **SBP** |  |
| **DBP** |  |
| **PULSE** |  |

## DAY_ _ _ _ _ _ _ _ _ .

| BLOOD SUGAR | INSULIN DOSE | GRAMS CARB | ACTIVITY |
|---|---|---|---|
|  |  |  |  |
|  |  |  |  |
|  |  |  |  |
|  |  |  |  |

**STRESS LEVELS** _ _ _ _ _ _ _ _ _ _ _ _

**WATER INTAKE** ♡ ♡ ♡ ♡ ♡ ♡

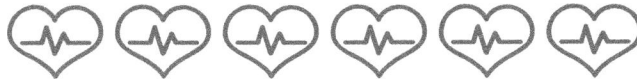

## EXERCISE AND DAILY ACTIVITIES

_____

_____

_____

_____

_____

_____

_____

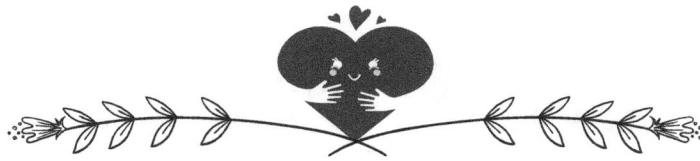

| DATE | |
|------|--|
| **TIME** | |
| **SBP** | |
| **DBP** | |
| **PULSE** | |

## DAY_ _ _ _ _ _ _ _ .

| BLOOD SUGAR | INSULIN DOSE | GRAMS CARB | ACTIVITY |
|-------------|--------------|------------|----------|
| | | | |
| | | | |
| | | | |
| | | | |

**STRESS LEVELS** _ _ _ _ _ _ _ _ _ _ _ _ _ _ _

**WATER INTAKE**

## EXERCISE AND DAILY ACTIVITIES

_____

_____

_____

_____

_____

_____

_____

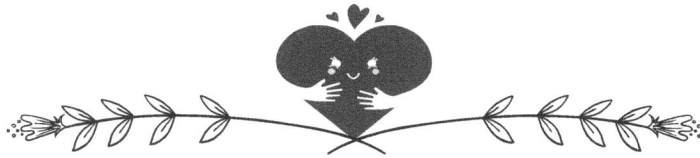

| DATE | |
|---|---|
| TIME | |
| SBP | |
| DBP | |
| PULSE | |

## DAY_ _ _ _ _ _ _ _ _ _ .

| BLOOD SUGAR | INSULIN DOSE | GRAMS CARB | ACTIVITY |
|---|---|---|---|
| | | | |
| | | | |
| | | | |
| | | | |

**STRESS LEVELS** _ _ _ _ _ _ _ _ _ _ _ _ _ _ _ _

**WATER INTAKE**

## EXERCISE AND DAILY ACTIVITIES

_____

_____

_____

_____

_____

_____

_____

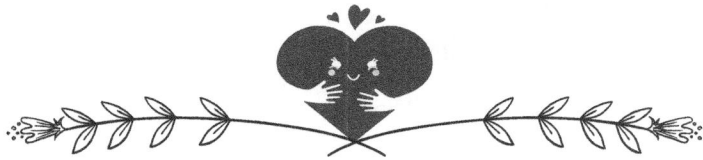

| DATE | |
|---|---|
| TIME | |
| SBP | |
| DBP | |
| PULSE | |

## DAY_ _ _ _ _ _ _ _ .

| BLOOD SUGAR | INSULIN DOSE | GRAMS CARB | ACTIVITY |
|---|---|---|---|
| | | | |
| | | | |
| | | | |
| | | | |

**STRESS LEVELS** _ _ _ _ _ _ _ _ _ _ _ _ _ _

**WATER INTAKE**

## EXERCISE AND DAILY ACTIVITIES

_____

_____

_____

_____

_____

_____

_____

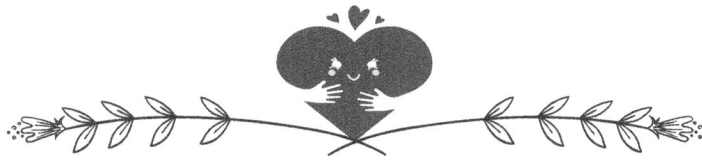

| | |
|---|---|
| **DATE** | |
| **TIME** | |
| **SBP** | |
| **DBP** | |
| **PULSE** | |

## DAY_ _ _ _ _ _ _ _ _ .

| BLOOD SUGAR | INSULIN DOSE | GRAMS CARB | ACTIVITY |
|---|---|---|---|
| | | | |
| | | | |
| | | | |
| | | | |

**STRESS LEVELS** _ _ _ _ _ _ _ _ _ _ _ _ _ _ _ _

**WATER INTAKE**

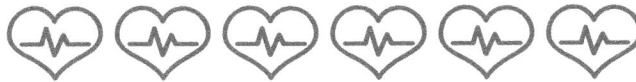

## EXERCISE AND DAILY ACTIVITIES

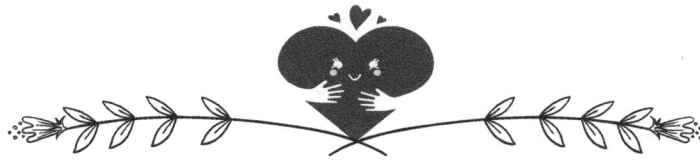

| DATE | |
|------|--|
| **TIME** | |
| **SBP** | |
| **DBP** | |
| **PULSE** | |

## DAY_ _ _ _ _ _ _ _ _ _ _ _ .

| BLOOD SUGAR | INSULIN DOSE | GRAMS CARB | ACTIVITY |
|-------------|--------------|------------|----------|
| | | | |
| | | | |
| | | | |
| | | | |

**STRESS LEVELS** _ _ _ _ _ _ _ _ _ _ _ _ _ _ _

**WATER INTAKE**

## EXERCISE AND DAILY ACTIVITIES

_____

_____

_____

_____

_____

_____

_____

_____

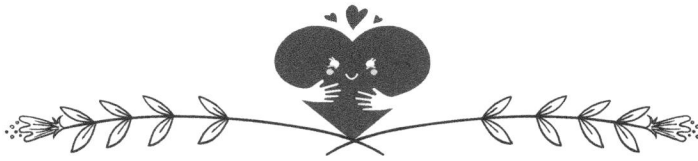

| DATE | |
|------|--|
| **TIME** | |
| **SBP** | |
| **DBP** | |
| **PULSE** | |

## DAY_ _ _ _ _ _ _ _ _ .

| BLOOD SUGAR | INSULIN DOSE | GRAMS CARB | ACTIVITY |
|-------------|--------------|------------|----------|
| | | | |
| | | | |
| | | | |
| | | | |

**STRESS LEVELS** _ _ _ _ _ _ _ _ _ _ _ _ _ _ _

**WATER INTAKE**

## EXERCISE AND DAILY ACTIVITIES

_____

_____

_____

_____

_____

_____

_____

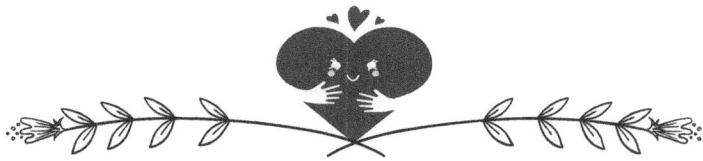

| DATE | |
|------|---|
| **TIME** | |
| **SBP** | |
| **DBP** | |
| **PULSE** | |

## DAY_ _ _ _ _ _ _ _ _ .

| BLOOD SUGAR | INSULIN DOSE | GRAMS CARB | ACTIVITY |
|-------------|--------------|------------|----------|
| | | | |
| | | | |
| | | | |
| | | | |

**STRESS LEVELS** _ _ _ _ _ _ _ _ _ _ _ _ _ _ _

**WATER INTAKE**

## EXERCISE AND DAILY ACTIVITIES

_____

_____

_____

_____

_____

_____

_____

_____

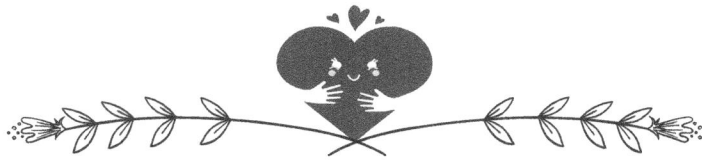

| DATE | |
|------|--|
| TIME | |
| SBP | |
| DBP | |
| PULSE | |

## DAY_ _ _ _ _ _ _ _ _ .

| BLOOD SUGAR | INSULIN DOSE | GRAMS CARB | ACTIVITY |
|-------------|--------------|------------|----------|
| | | | |
| | | | |
| | | | |
| | | | |

**STRESS LEVELS** _ _ _ _ _ _ _ _ _ _ _ _ _ _

**WATER INTAKE**

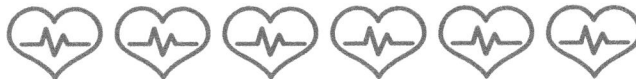

## EXERCISE AND DAILY ACTIVITIES

_____

_____

_____

_____

_____

_____

_____

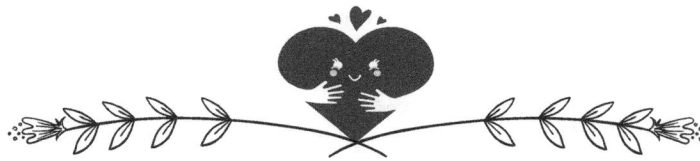

| DATE | |
| TIME | |
| SBP | |
| DBP | |
| PULSE | |

## DAY_ _ _ _ _ _ _ _ _ .

| BLOOD SUGAR | INSULIN DOSE | GRAMS CARB | ACTIVITY |
|---|---|---|---|
| | | | |
| | | | |
| | | | |
| | | | |

**STRESS LEVELS** _ _ _ _ _ _ _ _ _ _ _ _ _

**WATER INTAKE**

## EXERCISE AND DAILY ACTIVITIES

_____

_____

_____

_____

_____

_____

_____

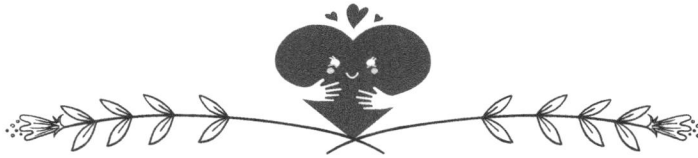

| DATE |  |
|---|---|
| TIME |  |
| SBP |  |
| DBP |  |
| PULSE |  |

## DAY_ _ _ _ _ _ _ _ _ _ .

| BLOOD SUGAR | INSULIN DOSE | GRAMS CARB | ACTIVITY |
|---|---|---|---|
|  |  |  |  |
|  |  |  |  |
|  |  |  |  |
|  |  |  |  |

**STRESS LEVELS** _ _ _ _ _ _ _ _ _ _ _ _ _ _ _

**WATER INTAKE**

## EXERCISE AND DAILY ACTIVITIES

_____

_____

_____

_____

_____

_____

_____

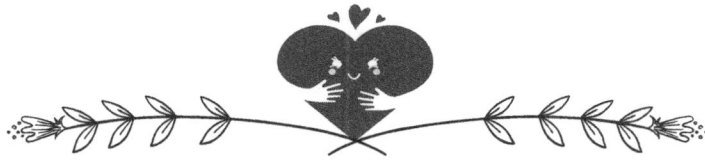

| DATE | |
|------|--|
| **TIME** | |
| **SBP** | |
| **DBP** | |
| **PULSE** | |

## DAY_ _ _ _ _ _ _ _ _ _ .

| BLOOD SUGAR | INSULIN DOSE | GRAMS CARB | ACTIVITY |
|-------------|--------------|------------|----------|
| | | | |
| | | | |
| | | | |
| | | | |

**STRESS LEVELS** _ _ _ _ _ _ _ _ _ _ _ _ _ _ _

**WATER INTAKE**

## EXERCISE AND DAILY ACTIVITIES

_____

_____

_____

_____

_____

_____

_____

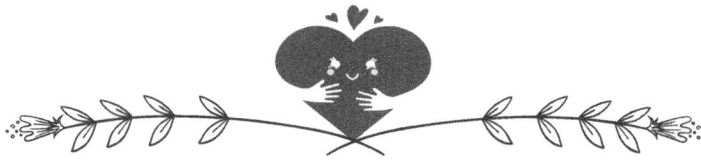

| DATE |  |
|------|--|

| TIME |  |
|------|--|

| SBP |  |
|-----|--|

| DBP |  |
|-----|--|

| PULSE |  |
|-------|--|

## DAY_ _ _ _ _ _ _ _ .

| BLOOD SUGAR | INSULIN DOSE | GRAMS CARB | ACTIVITY |
|-------------|--------------|------------|----------|
|  |  |  |  |
|  |  |  |  |
|  |  |  |  |
|  |  |  |  |

**STRESS LEVELS** _ _ _ _ _ _ _ _ _ _ _ _ _ _ _ _ _

**WATER INTAKE**

## EXERCISE AND DAILY ACTIVITIES

_____

_____

_____

_____

_____

_____

_____

_____

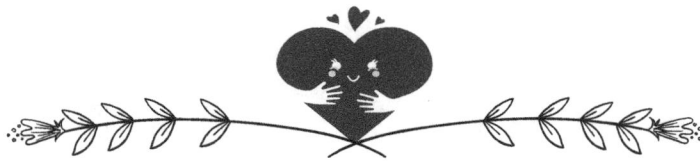

| DATE |  |
|------|--|
| **TIME** |  |
| **SBP** |  |
| **DBP** |  |
| **PULSE** |  |

## DAY_ _ _ _ _ _ _ _ .

| BLOOD SUGAR | INSULIN DOSE | GRAMS CARB | ACTIVITY |
|-------------|--------------|------------|----------|
|             |              |            |          |
|             |              |            |          |
|             |              |            |          |
|             |              |            |          |

**STRESS LEVELS** _ _ _ _ _ _ _ _ _ _ _ _ _ _ _ _ _

**WATER INTAKE** ♡ ♡ ♡ ♡ ♡ ♡

## EXERCISE AND DAILY ACTIVITIES

_____

_____

_____

_____

_____

_____

_____

_____

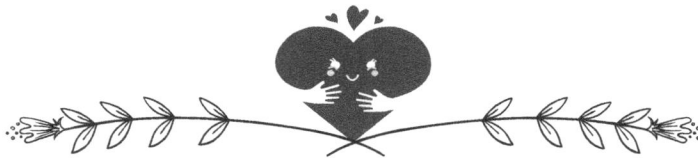

| DATE | |
|------|---|
| **TIME** | |
| **SBP** | |
| **DBP** | |
| **PULSE** | |

## DAY_ _ _ _ _ _ _ _ _ .

| BLOOD SUGAR | INSULIN DOSE | GRAMS CARB | ACTIVITY |
|-------------|--------------|-----------|----------|
| | | | |
| | | | |
| | | | |
| | | | |

**STRESS LEVELS** _ _ _ _ _ _ _ _ _ _ _ _ _ _

**WATER INTAKE**

## EXERCISE AND DAILY ACTIVITIES

_____

_____

_____

_____

_____

_____

_____

_____

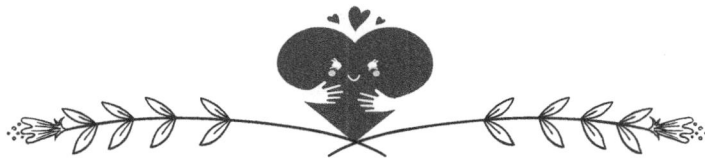

| DATE |  |
|------|--|
| TIME |  |
| SBP |  |
| DBP |  |
| PULSE |  |

## DAY _ _ _ _ _ _ _ _ .

| BLOOD SUGAR | INSULIN DOSE | GRAMS CARB | ACTIVITY |
|-------------|--------------|------------|----------|
|  |  |  |  |
|  |  |  |  |
|  |  |  |  |
|  |  |  |  |

**STRESS LEVELS** _ _ _ _ _ _ _ _ _ _ _ _ _ _ _ _

**WATER INTAKE**

## EXERCISE AND DAILY ACTIVITIES

_____

_____

_____

_____

_____

_____

_____

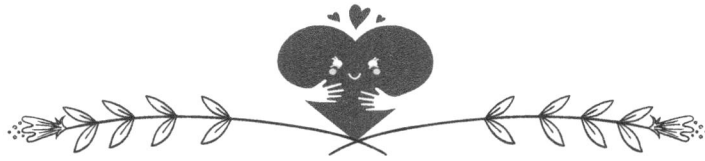

| DATE | |
|---|---|
| TIME | |
| SBP | |
| DBP | |
| PULSE | |

## DAY_ _ _ _ _ _ _ _ _ _ _ .

| BLOOD SUGAR | INSULIN DOSE | GRAMS CARB | ACTIVITY |
|---|---|---|---|
| | | | |
| | | | |
| | | | |
| | | | |

**STRESS LEVELS** _ _ _ _ _ _ _ _ _ _ _ _ _ _ _

**WATER INTAKE**

## EXERCISE AND DAILY ACTIVITIES

_____

_____

_____

_____

_____

_____

_____

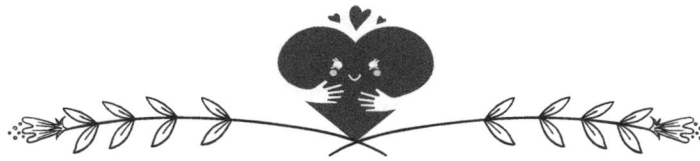

| DATE | |
|------|-|
| TIME | |
| SBP | |
| DBP | |
| PULSE | |

## DAY _ _ _ _ _ _ _ _ .

| BLOOD SUGAR | INSULIN DOSE | GRAMS CARB | ACTIVITY |
|-------------|--------------|-----------|----------|
| | | | |
| | | | |
| | | | |
| | | | |

**STRESS LEVELS** _ _ _ _ _ _ _ _ _ _ _ _ _ _ _

**WATER INTAKE**

## EXERCISE AND DAILY ACTIVITIES

_____

_____

_____

_____

_____

_____

_____

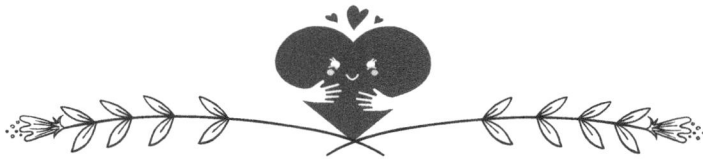

| DATE |  |
|------|--|
| **TIME** |  |
| **SBP** |  |
| **DBP** |  |
| **PULSE** |  |

## DAY_ _ _ _ _ _ _ _ _ _ .

| BLOOD SUGAR | INSULIN DOSE | GRAMS CARB | ACTIVITY |
|-------------|--------------|------------|----------|
|  |  |  |  |
|  |  |  |  |
|  |  |  |  |
|  |  |  |  |

**STRESS LEVELS** _ _ _ _ _ _ _ _ _ _ _ _ _ _ _

**WATER INTAKE**

## EXERCISE AND DAILY ACTIVITIES

_____

_____

_____

_____

_____

_____

_____

_____

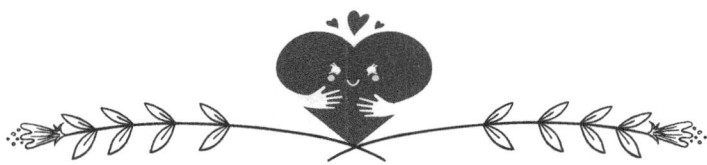

| DATE | |
| TIME | |
| SBP | |
| DBP | |
| PULSE | |

## DAY _ _ _ _ _ _ _ _ .

| BLOOD SUGAR | INSULIN DOSE | GRAMS CARB | ACTIVITY |
|---|---|---|---|
| | | | |
| | | | |
| | | | |
| | | | |

**STRESS LEVELS** _ _ _ _ _ _ _ _ _ _ _ _ _ _ _ _

**WATER INTAKE**

## EXERCISE AND DAILY ACTIVITIES

_____

_____

_____

_____

_____

_____

_____

_____

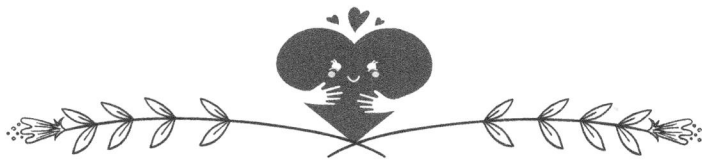

| DATE | |
|---|---|
| TIME | |
| SBP | |
| DBP | |
| PULSE | |

## DAY_ _ _ _ _ _ _ _ _ .

| BLOOD SUGAR | INSULIN DOSE | GRAMS CARB | ACTIVITY |
|---|---|---|---|
| | | | |
| | | | |
| | | | |
| | | | |

**STRESS LEVELS** _ _ _ _ _ _ _ _ _ _ _ _

**WATER INTAKE**

## EXERCISE AND DAILY ACTIVITIES

_____

_____

_____

_____

_____

_____

_____

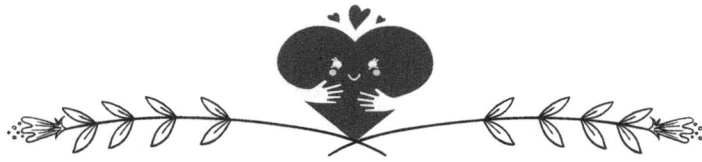

| DATE | |
| TIME | |
| SBP | |
| DBP | |
| PULSE | |

## DAY_ _ _ _ _ _ _ _ _ _ _ .

| BLOOD SUGAR | INSULIN DOSE | GRAMS CARB | ACTIVITY |
|---|---|---|---|
| | | | |
| | | | |
| | | | |
| | | | |

**STRESS LEVELS** _ _ _ _ _ _ _ _ _ _ _ _ _

**WATER INTAKE**

## EXERCISE AND DAILY ACTIVITIES

_____

_____

_____

_____

_____

_____

_____

_____

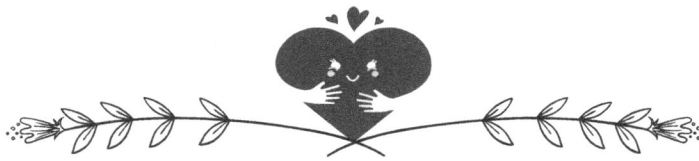

| DATE |  |
|------|--|

| TIME |  |
|------|--|

| SBP |  |
|-----|--|

| DBP |  |
|-----|--|

| PULSE |  |
|-------|--|

## DAY_ _ _ _ _ _ _ _ _ .

| BLOOD SUGAR | INSULIN DOSE | GRAMS CARB | ACTIVITY |
|-------------|--------------|------------|----------|
|  |  |  |  |
|  |  |  |  |
|  |  |  |  |
|  |  |  |  |

**STRESS LEVELS** _ _ _ _ _ _ _ _ _ _ _ _ _ _

**WATER INTAKE**  ♥ ♥ ♥ ♥ ♥ ♥

## EXERCISE AND DAILY ACTIVITIES

_____

_____

_____

_____

_____

_____

_____

_____

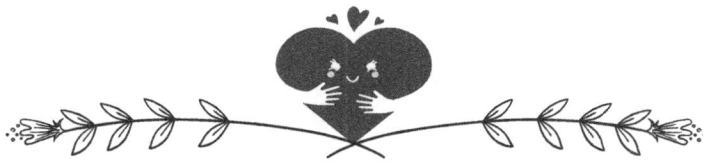

| DATE  |  |
|-------|--|
| TIME  |  |
| SBP   |  |
| DBP   |  |
| PULSE |  |

## DAY_ _ _ _ _ _ _ _ _ .

| BLOOD SUGAR | INSULIN DOSE | GRAMS CARB | ACTIVITY |
|-------------|--------------|------------|----------|
|             |              |            |          |
|             |              |            |          |
|             |              |            |          |
|             |              |            |          |

**STRESS LEVELS** _ _ _ _ _ _ _ _ _ _ _ _ _ _ _

**WATER INTAKE**

## EXERCISE AND DAILY ACTIVITIES

_____

_____

_____

_____

_____

_____

_____

_____

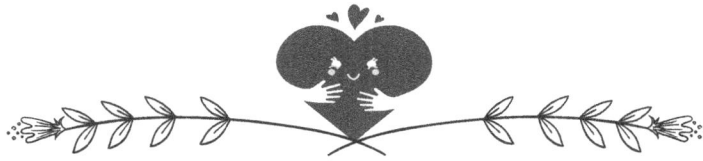

| DATE | |
|------|---|
| TIME | |
| SBP | |
| DBP | |
| PULSE | |

## DAY _ _ _ _ _ _ _ _ _ .

| BLOOD SUGAR | INSULIN DOSE | GRAMS CARB | ACTIVITY |
|-------------|--------------|------------|----------|
| | | | |
| | | | |
| | | | |
| | | | |

**STRESS LEVELS** _ _ _ _ _ _ _ _ _ _ _ _ _ _

**WATER INTAKE**

## EXERCISE AND DAILY ACTIVITIES

_____

_____

_____

_____

_____

_____

_____

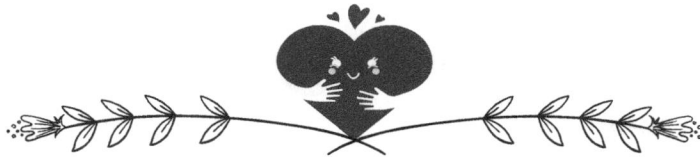

| DATE |  |
|------|--|
| TIME |  |
| SBP |  |
| DBP |  |
| PULSE |  |

## DAY_ _ _ _ _ _ _ _ .

| BLOOD SUGAR | INSULIN DOSE | GRAMS CARB | ACTIVITY |
|-------------|--------------|------------|----------|
|  |  |  |  |
|  |  |  |  |
|  |  |  |  |
|  |  |  |  |

**STRESS LEVELS** _ _ _ _ _ _ _ _ _ _ _ _ _ _

**WATER INTAKE**

## EXERCISE AND DAILY ACTIVITIES

_____

_____

_____

_____

_____

_____

_____

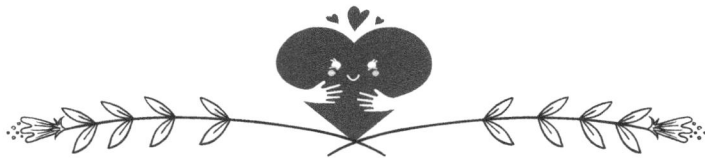

| DATE |  |
|------|--|
| **TIME** |  |
| **SBP** |  |
| **DBP** |  |
| **PULSE** |  |

## DAY_ _ _ _ _ _ _ _ _ _ .

| BLOOD SUGAR | INSULIN DOSE | GRAMS CARB | ACTIVITY |
|-------------|--------------|------------|----------|
|  |  |  |  |
|  |  |  |  |
|  |  |  |  |
|  |  |  |  |

**STRESS LEVELS** _ _ _ _ _ _ _ _ _ _ _ _ _ _

**WATER INTAKE**

## EXERCISE AND DAILY ACTIVITIES

_____

_____

_____

_____

_____

_____

_____

_____

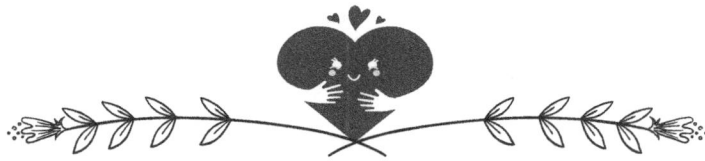

| DATE |  |
|------|--|

| TIME |  |
|------|--|

| SBP |  |
|-----|--|

| DBP |  |
|-----|--|

| PULSE |  |
|-------|--|

## DAY_ _ _ _ _ _ _ _.

| BLOOD SUGAR | INSULIN DOSE | GRAMS CARB | ACTIVITY |
|-------------|--------------|------------|----------|
|  |  |  |  |
|  |  |  |  |
|  |  |  |  |
|  |  |  |  |

**STRESS LEVELS** _ _ _ _ _ _ _ _ _ _ _ _ _ _

**WATER INTAKE**

## EXERCISE AND DAILY ACTIVITIES

_____

_____

_____

_____

_____

_____

_____

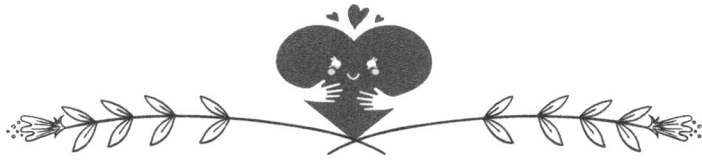

| DATE |  |
|------|--|
| **TIME** |  |
| **SBP** |  |
| **DBP** |  |
| **PULSE** |  |

## DAY_ _ _ _ _ _ _ _ .

| BLOOD SUGAR | INSULIN DOSE | GRAMS CARB | ACTIVITY |
|-------------|--------------|------------|----------|
|  |  |  |  |
|  |  |  |  |
|  |  |  |  |
|  |  |  |  |

**STRESS LEVELS** _ _ _ _ _ _ _ _ _ _ _ _ _ _ _ _

**WATER INTAKE**   ♡ ♡ ♡ ♡ ♡ ♡

## EXERCISE AND DAILY ACTIVITIES

_____

_____

_____

_____

_____

_____

_____

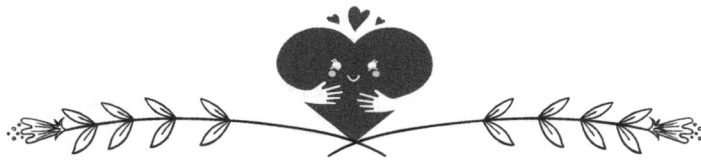

| DATE |  |
|------|--|
| TIME |  |
| SBP |  |
| DBP |  |
| PULSE |  |

## DAY _ _ _ _ _ _ _ .

| BLOOD SUGAR | INSULIN DOSE | GRAMS CARB | ACTIVITY |
|-------------|--------------|------------|----------|
|  |  |  |  |
|  |  |  |  |
|  |  |  |  |
|  |  |  |  |

**STRESS LEVELS** _ _ _ _ _ _ _ _ _ _ _ _ _ _ _

**WATER INTAKE**

## EXERCISE AND DAILY ACTIVITIES

_____

_____

_____

_____

_____

_____

_____

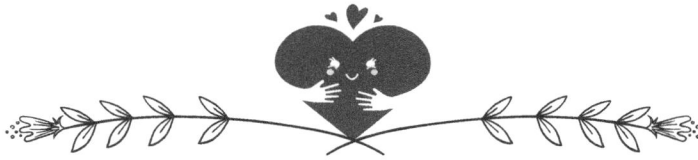

| DATE | |
|------|--|
| **TIME** | |
| **SBP** | |
| **DBP** | |
| **PULSE** | |

## DAY_ _ _ _ _ _ _ _ .

| BLOOD SUGAR | INSULIN DOSE | GRAMS CARB | ACTIVITY |
|-------------|--------------|-----------|----------|
|             |              |           |          |
|             |              |           |          |
|             |              |           |          |
|             |              |           |          |

**STRESS LEVELS** _ _ _ _ _ _ _ _ _ _ _ _ _ _ _ _

**WATER INTAKE**

## EXERCISE AND DAILY ACTIVITIES

_____

_____

_____

_____

_____

_____

_____

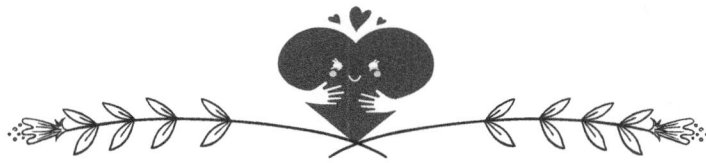

| DATE | |
|------|--|
| **TIME** | |
| **SBP** | |
| **DBP** | |
| **PULSE** | |

## DAY_ _ _ _ _ _ _ _ _ _ _ _ _ .

| BLOOD SUGAR | INSULIN DOSE | GRAMS CARB | ACTIVITY |
|-------------|--------------|------------|----------|
|             |              |            |          |
|             |              |            |          |
|             |              |            |          |
|             |              |            |          |

**STRESS LEVELS** _ _ _ _ _ _ _ _ _ _ _ _ _ _ _ _

**WATER INTAKE**

## EXERCISE AND DAILY ACTIVITIES

_____

_____

_____

_____

_____

_____

_____

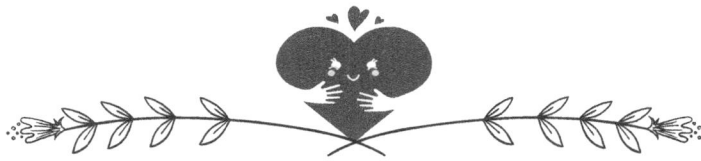

| DATE |  |
|------|--|
| **TIME** |  |
| **SBP** |  |
| **DBP** |  |
| **PULSE** |  |

## DAY_ _ _ _ _ _ _ _ .

| BLOOD SUGAR | INSULIN DOSE | GRAMS CARB | ACTIVITY |
|-------------|--------------|------------|----------|
|  |  |  |  |
|  |  |  |  |
|  |  |  |  |
|  |  |  |  |

**STRESS LEVELS** _ _ _ _ _ _ _ _ _ _ _ _ _ _ _ _ _

**WATER INTAKE**

## EXERCISE AND DAILY ACTIVITIES

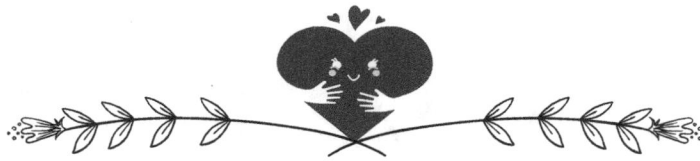

| DATE | |
|------|--|
| TIME | |
| SBP | |
| DBP | |
| PULSE | |

## DAY_ _ _ _ _ _ _ _ _ _ _ .

| BLOOD SUGAR | INSULIN DOSE | GRAMS CARB | ACTIVITY |
|-------------|--------------|-----------|----------|
|             |              |           |          |
|             |              |           |          |
|             |              |           |          |
|             |              |           |          |

**STRESS LEVELS** _ _ _ _ _ _ _ _ _ _ _ _ _ _

**WATER INTAKE**

## EXERCISE AND DAILY ACTIVITIES

_____

_____

_____

_____

_____

_____

_____

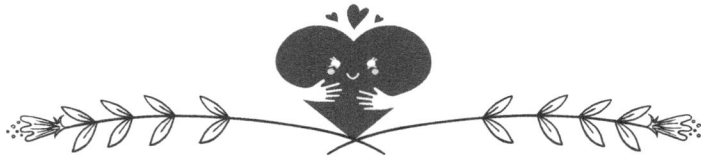

| DATE |  |
|------|--|
| **TIME** | |
| **SBP** | |
| **DBP** | |
| **PULSE** | |

## DAY_ _ _ _ _ _ _ _ _ _ .

| BLOOD SUGAR | INSULIN DOSE | GRAMS CARB | ACTIVITY |
|-------------|--------------|-----------|----------|
| | | | |
| | | | |
| | | | |
| | | | |

**STRESS LEVELS** _ _ _ _ _ _ _ _ _ _ _ _ _ _ _ _ _

**WATER INTAKE**

## EXERCISE AND DAILY ACTIVITIES

_____

_____

_____

_____

_____

_____

_____

_____

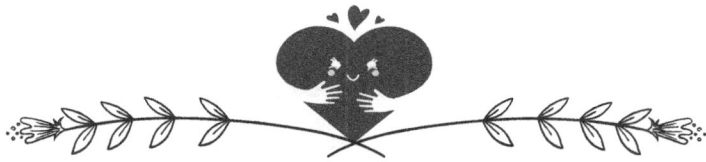

| DATE | |
|------|---|
| **TIME** | |
| **SBP** | |
| **DBP** | |
| **PULSE** | |

## DAY_ _ _ _ _ _ _ _ _ .

| BLOOD SUGAR | INSULIN DOSE | GRAMS CARB | ACTIVITY |
|-------------|--------------|------------|----------|
| | | | |
| | | | |
| | | | |
| | | | |

**STRESS LEVELS** _ _ _ _ _ _ _ _ _ _ _ _ _ _ _

**WATER INTAKE**

## EXERCISE AND DAILY ACTIVITIES

_____

_____

_____

_____

_____

_____

_____

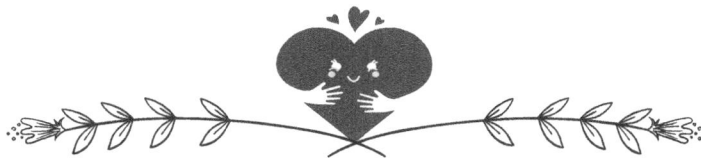

| DATE  |  |
|-------|--|
| TIME  |  |
| SBP   |  |
| DBP   |  |
| PULSE |  |

## DAY_ _ _ _ _ _ _ _ _ .

| BLOOD SUGAR | INSULIN DOSE | GRAMS CARB | ACTIVITY |
|-------------|--------------|------------|----------|
|             |              |            |          |
|             |              |            |          |
|             |              |            |          |
|             |              |            |          |

**STRESS LEVELS** _ _ _ _ _ _ _ _ _ _ _ _ _ _

**WATER INTAKE**

## EXERCISE AND DAILY ACTIVITIES

_____

_____

_____

_____

_____

_____

_____

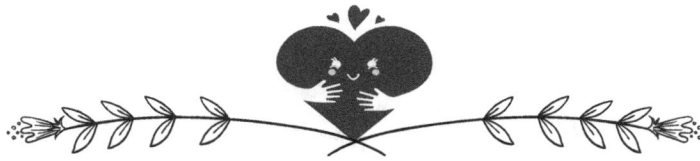

| DATE | |
|------|---|
| TIME | |
| SBP | |
| DBP | |
| PULSE | |

## DAY_ _ _ _ _ _ _ _ _ _ _ .

| BLOOD SUGAR | INSULIN DOSE | GRAMS CARB | ACTIVITY |
|-------------|--------------|-----------|----------|
| | | | |
| | | | |
| | | | |
| | | | |

**STRESS LEVELS** _ _ _ _ _ _ _ _ _ _ _ _ _

**WATER INTAKE**

## EXERCISE AND DAILY ACTIVITIES

_____

_____

_____

_____

_____

_____

_____

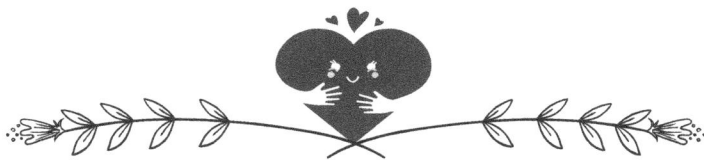

| DATE |  |
|------|--|
| TIME |  |
| SBP |  |
| DBP |  |
| PULSE |  |

## DAY_ _ _ _ _ _ _ _ _ .

| BLOOD SUGAR | INSULIN DOSE | GRAMS CARB | ACTIVITY |
|-------------|--------------|-----------|----------|
|             |              |           |          |
|             |              |           |          |
|             |              |           |          |
|             |              |           |          |

**STRESS LEVELS** _ _ _ _ _ _ _ _ _ _ _ _ _ _ _ _ _ _

**WATER INTAKE**

## EXERCISE AND DAILY ACTIVITIES

_____

_____

_____

_____

_____

_____

_____

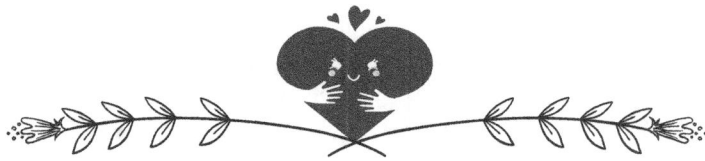

| DATE | |
|---|---|
| TIME | |
| SBP | |
| DBP | |
| PULSE | |

## DAY _ _ _ _ _ _ _ _ _ .

| BLOOD SUGAR | INSULIN DOSE | GRAMS CARB | ACTIVITY |
|---|---|---|---|
| | | | |
| | | | |
| | | | |
| | | | |

**STRESS LEVELS** _ _ _ _ _ _ _ _ _ _ _ _ _ _ _ _

**WATER INTAKE**

## EXERCISE AND DAILY ACTIVITIES

_____

_____

_____

_____

_____

_____

_____

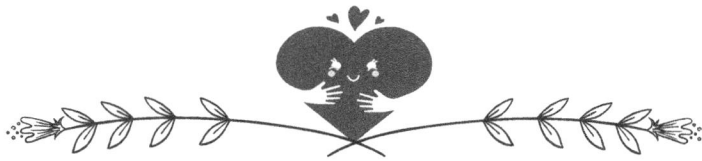

| DATE | |
| TIME | |
| SBP | |
| DBP | |
| PULSE | |

## DAY_ _ _ _ _ _ _ _ _ .

| BLOOD SUGAR | INSULIN DOSE | GRAMS CARB | ACTIVITY |
|---|---|---|---|
| | | | |
| | | | |
| | | | |
| | | | |

**STRESS LEVELS** _ _ _ _ _ _ _ _ _ _ _ _ _ _ _ _

**WATER INTAKE**

## EXERCISE AND DAILY ACTIVITIES

_____

_____

_____

_____

_____

_____

_____

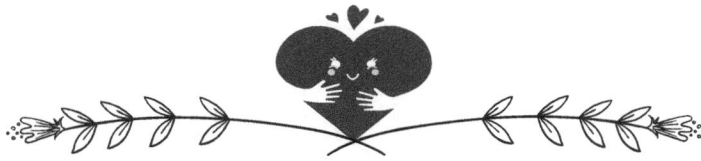

| DATE | |
| --- | --- |
| TIME | |
| SBP | |
| DBP | |
| PULSE | |

## DAY_ _ _ _ _ _ _ _ .

| BLOOD SUGAR | INSULIN DOSE | GRAMS CARB | ACTIVITY |
| --- | --- | --- | --- |
| | | | |
| | | | |
| | | | |
| | | | |

**STRESS LEVELS** _ _ _ _ _ _ _ _ _ _ _ _ _ _ _ _

**WATER INTAKE**

## EXERCISE AND DAILY ACTIVITIES

_____

_____

_____

_____

_____

_____

_____

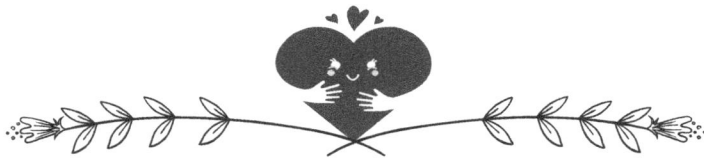

| DATE |  |
|---|---|
| TIME |  |
| SBP |  |
| DBP |  |
| PULSE |  |

## DAY_ _ _ _ _ _ _ _ _ .

| BLOOD SUGAR | INSULIN DOSE | GRAMS CARB | ACTIVITY |
|---|---|---|---|
|  |  |  |  |
|  |  |  |  |
|  |  |  |  |
|  |  |  |  |

**STRESS LEVELS** _ _ _ _ _ _ _ _ _ _ _ _ _ _ _ _ _

**WATER INTAKE**

## EXERCISE AND DAILY ACTIVITIES

_____

_____

_____

_____

_____

_____

_____

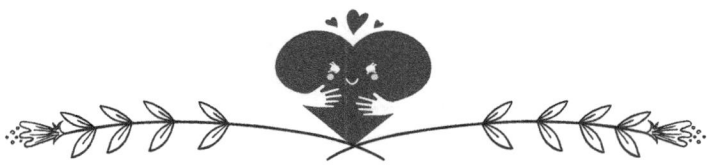

| DATE | |
|---|---|

| TIME | |
|---|---|

| SBP | |
|---|---|

| DBP | |
|---|---|

| PULSE | |
|---|---|

# DAY_ _ _ _ _ _ _ .

| BLOOD SUGAR | INSULIN DOSE | GRAMS CARB | ACTIVITY |
|---|---|---|---|
| | | | |
| | | | |
| | | | |
| | | | |

**STRESS LEVELS** _ _ _ _ _ _ _ _ _ _ _ _ _ _

**WATER INTAKE**

## EXERCISE AND DAILY ACTIVITIES

_____

_____

_____

_____

_____

_____

_____

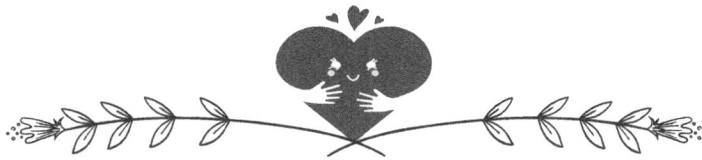

| DATE | |
|---|---|

| TIME | |
|---|---|

| SBP | |
|---|---|

| DBP | |
|---|---|

| PULSE | |
|---|---|

## DAY_ _ _ _ _ _ _ _ _ _ .

| BLOOD SUGAR | INSULIN DOSE | GRAMS CARB | ACTIVITY |
|---|---|---|---|
| | | | |
| | | | |
| | | | |
| | | | |

**STRESS LEVELS** _ _ _ _ _ _ _ _ _ _ _ _ _ _ _ _ _

**WATER INTAKE**

## EXERCISE AND DAILY ACTIVITIES

_____

_____

_____

_____

_____

_____

_____

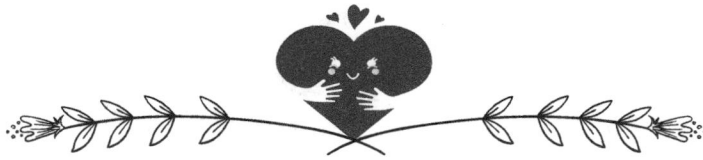

| DATE |  |
|---|---|
| TIME |  |
| SBP |  |
| DBP |  |
| PULSE |  |

## DAY_ _ _ _ _ _ _ _ _ _ _ .

| BLOOD SUGAR | INSULIN DOSE | GRAMS CARB | ACTIVITY |
|---|---|---|---|
|  |  |  |  |
|  |  |  |  |
|  |  |  |  |
|  |  |  |  |

**STRESS LEVELS** _ _ _ _ _ _ _ _ _ _ _ _ _ _ _

**WATER INTAKE**

## EXERCISE AND DAILY ACTIVITIES

_____

_____

_____

_____

_____

_____

_____

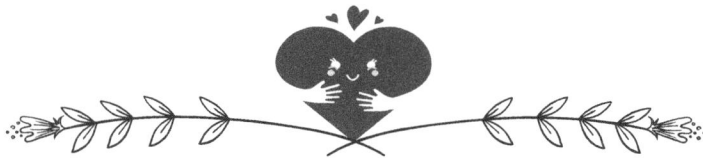

| DATE |  |
|---|---|
| **TIME** | |
| **SBP** | |
| **DBP** | |
| **PULSE** | |

## DAY_ _ _ _ _ _ _ _ _ .

| BLOOD SUGAR | INSULIN DOSE | GRAMS CARB | ACTIVITY |
|---|---|---|---|
| | | | |
| | | | |
| | | | |
| | | | |

**STRESS LEVELS** _ _ _ _ _ _ _ _ _ _ _ _ _ _

**WATER INTAKE**

## EXERCISE AND DAILY ACTIVITIES

_____

_____

_____

_____

_____

_____

_____

www.ingramcontent.com/pod-product-compliance
Lightning Source LLC
Chambersburg PA
CBHW081241220326
41597CB00023BA/4340

* 9 7 8 1 8 0 3 8 5 9 9 2 7 *